THE TURNAROUND IMPERATIVE

A Leader's Guide
for Survival in a
Turbulent Health
Care Environment

BY

Victor A. Cocowitch, MPH, and Kevin M. Fickenscher, MD, FACPE

American College of Physician Executives
4890 West Kennedy Boulevard • Suite 200 • Tampa, Florida 33609
813/287-2000

ISBN: 0-924674-37-7

Library of Congress Card Number: 95-79896

Printed in the United States of America by
Hillsboro Printing, Tampa, Florida

Dedicated to
The Lafite Four
and
Dawn and Sandi.

FOREWORD

Here is a practical guide for survival in a turbulent health care environment. I like this book. It is chockful of practical suggestions. It is well organized, clearly written, and a joy to read.

I have never been in a tsunami, but the authors, Victor Cocowitch and Kevin Fickenscher, have chosen an excellent metaphor for what is now appearing on the health care horizon. Change is increasing at an increasing rate. The old order is dying. The new is about to be born. We are entering a dynamic, high-threat, high-opportunity period. We are in-between the old and the new, the known and the unknown, the possible and the yet to be conceived. What a time to be alive! What a time to be in health care! The decisions we make in the next five years will cast a shadow for the next century.

I recommend this book for leaders of all health care organizations. It provides an excellent review of changing health care trends. Even better, it offers a practical guide on what to do about them. In many ways, *The Turnaround Imperative* is a survival manual for the remainder of the '90s and a thrival manual for the beginning of the 21st Century.

The authors describe The Change Continuum and its three major historical progressions: (1) Development (1970s), (2) Strategic (1980s), and (3) Transformational (1990s and beyond). The three progressions are then contrasted and compared. I find this analysis very useful. It provides a nice summary of what has been, now is, and soon will be happening in health care. It is both historical and predictive.

In addition to their perspectives on turnarounds, the authors discuss six key principles: (1) simultaneity, (2) rapidity, (3) complexity, (4) uncertainty, (5) management by intuition, and (6) leader objectivity. Now, I agree with all six principles, but imagine my surprise at their statement of the fifth one, management by intuition. Victor and Kevin are in a class by themselves in their recognition of this key variable in effective management. Most management books are too timid to discuss intuition. These authors not only recognize it; they suggest how to manage it. Tsunami or not, Victor and Kevin are clearly breaking new water with this important observation.

The Turnaround Imperative not only makes important an statement, it encourages reflection. Note the insightful questions it asks throughout the book. These are the same questions an expensive consultant would ask when visiting your organization. Please attempt to answer these questions. Better yet, take them to your board, medical staff, or management meetings as a discussion agenda. I am convinced the universe is only an answer. There are no questions in the universe. It is answers. It answers only the questions you ask. What happens if you ask the wrong questions? You got it—they are answered. *The Turnaround Imperative* asks the right questions. Listen for the answers.

I like computers. That may explain why I like *The Turnaround Imperative*. It is interactive and provides a graphic interface. Look at al the charts, graphs, tables, listings, and other visual devices. This is a user-friendly book. Pay special attention to what is printed in the boxes. These messages are succinct and pointed. Like "point and click" on your computer program, they will take you places.

You can also use *The Turnaround Imperative* as a guidebook for formulation of your organization's strategic plan. It provides a comprehensive conceptual framework for your thinking. It covers the waterfront and also indicates the way to higher ground. Just the thing to know in a tsunami.

In summary, you are in for a treat. Oh, I just noticed, the tide seems to be rapidly going out. I wonder what that means.

Leland R. Kaiser, PhD
Kaiser & Associates
Brighton, Colorado
January 5, 1996

PREFACE

How did this book come about? It all started on the back of a napkin. We were together back in 1989 and discussing whether or not an obvious turnaround situation deserved consideration as a career opportunity. Why not dive in? It seemed like an interesting challenge. Besides, the combination of an organizational development expert and a physician executive leader in health care seemed like a winning combination.

The turnaround experience was something else! On the second day, Kevin called Vic and said: "I think I've made a major, career-limiting mistake! Help!" And so began a process that we later came to call "surfing the tsunami." The challenges, the frustrations, and the opportunities in surfing tsunamis are a new dimension in health care. This book is a testament to those situations where *The Turnaround Imperative* is the only option.

Who is the audience? There are many people who will benefit from a book about turnarounds in health care. We believe that those who find themselves in a turnaround situation will be required to create a new organizational entity or structure out of an existing one. The difficulty is that, too frequently, the existing structure is no longer applicable to the times. Such is the dilemma of health care in the 1990s. The foundations of our nation's health care system are being eroded by tsunami after tsunami.

The major audience for *The Turnaround Imperative* is the leaders in health care organizations, such as senior administrators and managers, members of boards of directors, and physician executives. These are the individuals who will be leading the changes that are imminent in health care. Others who will benefit include providers of various types and persuasions, human resource professionals, organizational development and systems consultants, and educators.

What makes this book unique? First, the book is a focused discussion about turnarounds in health care. As we surveyed the literature of the past several years, it was obvious that little had been added in recent years about turnaround situations, and virtually nothing had been written about the phenomenon of turnarounds in health care settings.

Second, the book is not one person's perspective on turnarounds in health care. Rather, it represents a compilation of thinking by a team of two individuals with different ideas and thoughts on the turnaround process. Kevin M. Fickenscher, MD, is a physician executive/leader who has lived in the trenches of a turnaround situation. Vic Cocowitch is an organizational development expert with a wealth of experience in consulting with organizations at different stages in turnaround situations.

Third, the book is based on experiences and is an attempt to provide our colleagues in health care with a practical guide on how best to deal with a turnaround, not a textbook about turnarounds. It is not the definitive analysis of turnarounds, nor is it intended to be one. Rather, we believe that there is no singular solution for turnaround situations. Turnarounds, by their very nature, require composite and global thinking where the response to each situation requires a unique approach derived from a plethora of possibilities.

How do you use this book? The book can be read in one sitting of four hours (easily!) or in snippets over several weeks. We have attempted to construct a book that will be useful and not gather dust. Too many contemporary books on business aren't that useful because of the weight of detail. We have attempted to provide sufficient detail and yet keep the material simple. Along that line of thinking, we encourage you to keep it close at hand, in a drawer, under some papers, or in your favorite hideaway at home for those times when you're rethinking your turnaround strategy. Remember, turnarounds are as much about process (how to proceed) as they are about content (what to do). We hope this book will enhance your survival as a turnaround artist.

Who needs to be acknowledged? We simply couldn't have done this project without the support of Dawn and Sandi—our spouses—our friends, our buddies, and our most demanding critics! Not only did they tolerate our time together, but they also encouraged us where others questioned the concept.

There came a time in the writing of *The Turnaround Imperative* when we realized we needed help. The finances of turnarounds are an essential part of a successful effort. Ray Barton III provided a valuable addendum to the book when he agreed to write the chapter on finances. He has a wealth of experience in the trenches of health care turnarounds and is particularly adept on financial strategies. Without his contributions, the book would not have the required depth. We thank him!

Charlie and Edie Seashore have helped us both in good times and tough times. They continue to be—in our lives—people of infinite wisdom about how to approach complex change and seem to be able to share it with humor and insight. They uniquely help leaders integrate both personal and professional considerations in their work. Such help is absolutely essential in the formative stages of a turnaround. We need to remember that organizations are driven by people and leaders, not by some inhuman engine in the basement someplace. Charlie and Edie have made that idea a reality for us.

We also want to thank Theodore Wille, Robert Van Hook, and Suzanne Eichorn, three friends and professional colleagues. Ted is one of the clearest thinking leaders we know on the evolving nature of managed care in the nation. Bob is in the thick of helping to formulate the evolving nature of our reforming health care system. Suzanne provided us with unique insights about the complex change evolving in the health care field. Their wisdom, extensive experience and support have been invaluable assets in writing about *The Turnaround Imperative*.

Finally, the support and encouragement of Wes Curry at the American College of Physician Executives has been a driving force in helping us to finish the book. Deadlines do make a difference, especially when there is the press of other responsibilities and tasks.

Vic Cocowitch, MPH   *Kevin Fickenscher, MD, FACPE*
Chapel Hill, North Carolina   *Milwaukee, Wisconsin*
January 5, 1996   *January 5, 1996*

ABOUT THE AUTHORS

Vic Cocowitch, MPH, has extensive management and consulting experience in the health care industry. He has an educational background in both health administration and organizational development. Vic attended the University of North Carolina, where he received an undergraduate degree in economics and his master's degree in public health administration. He also completed the Johns Hopkins University Program in Organizational and Community Systems. He is a faculty member of the NTL Institute for Applied Behavioral Sciences and the Center for Creative Leadership.

Vic's consulting practice uniquely combines his health care management expertise with skills in change and strategic management, human relations, and group facilitation. His previous management positions have included senior level staff positions in health care associations, hospitals, and staff/IPA model HMOs.

He has consulted with a wide spectrum of clients, including numerous national health care associations, health professions education institutions, hospitals, managed care plans, and health care agencies. Central to his work are the themes of assisting senior level managers and boards to plan their organizations' futures and supporting their roles as change agents to ensure viability.

Vic's consulting role involves turnaround management, strategic planning, team building, board development, large-scale culture change, conflict resolution, and total quality or reengineering efforts. He is also a nationally qualified user and trainer with the Myers-Briggs Type Indicator (MBTI).

He has served on a variety of national boards and advisory committees for foundations and health care organizations. He thinks he is a better chef than Kevin. He is a better golfer.

Kevin Fickenscher, MD, FACPE, in addition to his training in health care, has directed a turnaround effort. He frequently consults with organizations on health care issues and has worked with small hospitals, large tertiary care centers, physician groups, universities, systems, regional and national organizations, state and federal governments, foundations, and other entities interested in the future of the American health care system. Kevin's areas of expertise relate to strategic planning, the future of health care, integration of health care delivery systems, medical education, community development, and leadership.

Kevin graduated from the University of North Dakota School of Medicine in 1978. Following graduation, he obtained two years of family medicine training at the Residency Program in Social Medicine at Montefiore Hospital and Medical Center, Bronx, New York, and completed his last two years of training with the

Department of Family Medicine through the University of North Dakota while concurrently developing a rural health program. He obtained his Family Practice Board certification in 1982.

In his first professional challenge as a physician executive, he organized and developed The Center for Rural Health at the University of North Dakota. The Center is a nationally prominent program dedicated to rural health service, research, and policy analysis. Kevin is also a noted leader on issues related to rural health and Past President of the National Rural Health Association. Subsequently, he served as the Assistant Dean and President/CEO of the Michigan State University Kalamazoo Center for Medical Studies, a campus of the MSU College of Human Medicine.

He is presently Senior Vice President and Chief Medical Officer of Aurora Health Care, an integrated health care system based in Milwaukee, Wisconsin. He is the primary liaison with medical and health practitioners in the region, an active participant in strategic planning for the corporation, and the organizer of effective physician-governance-management interfaces.

Kevin is certified by the American Board of Medical Management and is a Fellow of the American College of Physician Executives. He also retains membership in the American College of Healthcare Executives, the American Academy of Family Physicians, the National Rural Health Association, and various other professional organizations. He is a Past Chairman of the Board of Trustees for Catholic Health Corporation, a multi-institutional organization with more than 100 facilities in 14 states based in Omaha, Nebraska; a member of the Board of Trustees of the Sisters of Charity Health Care System, a multi-institutional system based in Cincinnati, Ohio; a member of the Board of Stewardship for Catholic Health Initiatives based in Denver, Colorado; and a member of the Healthcare Forum Board of Directors.

In addition to his academic and management interests, Kevin is very involved in health policy at the local, state, and national levels as a noted expert on health care systems. Among other recognitions for leadership, Kevin was the recipient of a Kellogg National Fellowship, a Regional Finalist for the White House Fellowship, and the Healthcare Forum-Korn/Ferry International Emerging Leader in Healthcare for 1991. More recently, he served as a member of the Health Professions Advisory Group to President Clinton's Task Force on Health Care Reform. He enjoys food more than Vic and is the penultimate duffer.

TABLE OF CONTENTS

A Metaphor...The Beginnings: Lessons from Tsunami Waves
The tsunami is a metaphor for the changes that will roll over the United States health care system for many years to come. These waves of change are moving quickly toward their destination and have been largely ignored by too many leaders in the health care industry. The lessons of the tsunami are an important foundation for understanding the future by the health care leader.

What Is a Turnaround?: The Ultimate Change Experience—Surfing the Tsunami
The chapter provides a technical description of the turnaround and reviews change responses relevant to understanding a turnaround. The six key principles essential to a turnaround are highlighted.

Why Turnarounds?: The Change Imperative in Health Care—The Tsunami Warning
Turnarounds must be considered in an environmental context. The environmental trends affecting the American health care system are considered, and the reasons for an increase in turnaround situations in health care during the coming decade are outlined.

CHAPTER I

A Metaphor...
The Beginnings

*"All of a sudden...the ship went up, or maybe I went down.
The dock just fell in and I saw this big comber wave full
of timber rolling in way above me."*

Seaman Ted Pedersen
Tsunami Survivor
Good Friday, 1964[1]

Lessons from Tsunami Waves

In the search for a way to describe the many changes in health care, water seems to be a common theme. We've all heard the predictions about the white water that will be sweeping the health care industry. Then, as if white water wasn't enough, it became *permanent white water*.[2] Another author has described the environment as a process of riding the waves of change. He states:

> In developing managerial competencies, it is not enough to look at what excellent organizations and managers are already doing. It is also necessary to be proactive in relation to the future: to anticipate some of the changes that are likely to occur and to position organizations and their members to address these new challenges effectively.[3]

We even have the federal government getting into the water analogy business, with the use of *safe harbor* designations as a definition for activities that can be safely pursued as joint initiatives between hospitals and physicians.

White water, permanent white water, waves, and safe harbors are all good analogies for the current situation in health care. Wherever there is water, there are inevitably waves. But we feel a better metaphor for many of today's health care institutions is the tsunami. Tsunami, a Japanese term, means *harbor* wave, relating to the wave's destination, not its origin. The tsunami is an oceanic wave that emanates from a specific source, is not random, and is not related to wind. It's the largest type of wave known to mankind—when it hits its destination. At sea, the tsunami often goes unnoticed. Unlike the ordinary wave, which, through its continuous action, rocks us about and erodes our confidence, the tsunami sweeps over the shoreline and destroys everything in its path. After a tsunami hits, little remains the same.

Lots of waves are pounding on the shores of the health care industry. Change in health care is an imperative. Regardless of the origin of the environmental changes in health care, they are now beginning to crash down like the tsunami at the institutional and provider levels. Many organizations will be affected by the coming health reform initiative, even those not directly at the shoreline of change. The primary focus of change will be directed at hospitals, physician groups, insurance companies, and local community health care systems. As a result, we can anticipate substantial restructuring of health care in communities across the nation as they respond to the repeated tsunami waves of change in business practices, alliances, and reform initiatives.

 Whatever the cause, the tsunami starts with a sudden jolt or tremor that displaces the water.

Although the changes in health care can be attributed to many factors, there is an overriding issue of national concern that serves as the nidus for the debate on health care reform. The impact of the global economy on the United States, although not well understood, should not be underestimated as a major factor in stimulating the health reform debate.

Participation in the global economy requires maximal efficiency and productivity if one's products are to be competitive. Unlike the years following World War II, when the U.S. economy was essentially the only game in town, our goods and services must compete with those of countries throughout the world, whether it's cars from Japan, shoes from Thailand, wine from Chile, or corn from Mexico. Not only must we keep quality up, but also costs must be kept down. As a result, every addition to the cost of goods and services produced in this country must be scrutinized.

As business has squeezed the costs of production down, it has become increasingly apparent that the marginal contribution of health care costs to the overall cost of goods and services produced in the United States is not inconsequential. In fact, it can be easily argued that the margin of difference contributed by health care to the costs of U.S. produced goods and services will determine, in many cases, whether or not the products and services are competitive in the world marketplace.

Because health care expenditures as a percentage of Gross Domestic Product (GDP) for the United States far outstrip those of the rest of the world (see the figure on page 00), the United States must make up for these excess costs (on a comparative basis) through efficiency and productivity gains. The major problem for American business is that, because of the continuous ratcheting down process in

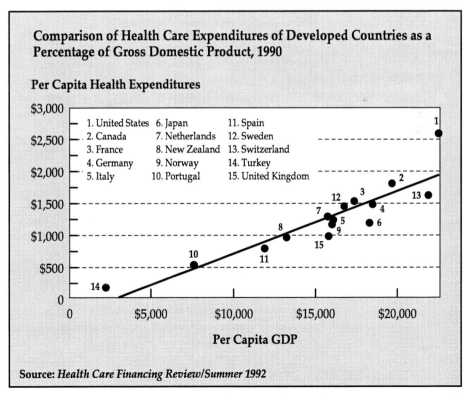

Comparison of Health Care Expenditures of Developed Countries as a Percentage of Gross Domestic Product, 1990

Per Capita Health Expenditures

1. United States 6. Japan   11. Spain
2. Canada   7. Netherlands 12. Sweden
3. France   8. New Zealand 13. Switzerland
4. Germany   9. Norway   14. Turkey
5. Italy   10. Portugal   15. United Kingdom

Per Capita GDP

Source: *Health Care Financing Review/Summer 1992*

Thera: The Origin of Atlantis?

"The legend of Atlantis has long fascinated the west. The story of an island empire that sank into the sea in a single dire catastrophe was recorded by Plato. The modern theory of plate tectonics forbids the idea that a large island could actually have sunk in the Atlantic. Scientists now believe the civilization was Crete, the island Thera (also spelled Thira, and now known as Santorini), and that the explosion, Krakatoa-like, happened about 1450 B.C. The explosion must have been truly enormous. An island 10 or 12 miles (16-18 kilometers) across was turned in an instant from a 5000 foot (1500 meters) peak into a lagoon. Such an explosion—four or five times that of Krakatoa—could have sent a huge ash fall and a massive tsunami across the 70 miles to Crete, as well as burying its own major city, Akrotiri, now being unearthed."[4]

global competition, U.S. producers of goods and services find it increasingly difficult to wring ever more efficiency and productivity out of the system.

It is highly unlikely that the global economic developments of the past decade will disappear anytime soon. Therefore, it becomes even more of a societal imperative to control our nation's *elective* (i.e., nonentitlement) expenditures. Health care, like education and the military, is essentially an elective expenditure of society.

The global economy has everything to do with the future of health care in the United States. From the perspective of *The Turnaround Imperative,* it is central to the discussion of why health care reform has become not only an economic imperative, but also a societal imperative.

The health care institutions of our nation have been dominated by an "it'll-never-happen-here" mentality. Hospitals and physicians, in particular, seem to possess a predominant attitude that change will never occur. It's just another point of discussion in the ongoing debate. Such an attitude creates the perfect environment for the tsunami. By ignoring the warnings, we are preparing for the inevitable destruction of the tsunami.

 The tsunami that hits shore started someplace far away and often is not fully appreciated until it hits shore.

The trends are evident throughout the nation. In California, integrated delivery networks are sweeping the health care landscape. In Minnesota, an integrated delivery system has emerged as a dominant player in the metropolitan Minneapolis, area, with a 25 percent market share. In Wisconsin, the strategic alliance of Dean Health Systems (a 450-physician multispecialty group) and Aurora Health Care (a regional hospital system with a 350-physician multispecialty group) is changing the face of health care delivery in the Upper Midwest.

Large multifacility systems have become dominate players in the health care marketplace. Who would have thought one year ago that strategic plans for some of these behemoths would consider options to disband? Did we hear it right—the standard bearer of academic medicine, the University of Washington Medical Center, is actively pursuing integration with private practices and groups throughout the Seattle area! And the consolidation goes on. In Albuquerque, New Mexico, the marketplace has gone from a large number of independent hospitals to four dominant systems in the space of 10 years! These are mere examples of trends happening all over the country.

These responses are pragmatic rejoinders to the very real cost control demands of American business. It is clear that the trends toward consolidation, collaboration, and integration will continue. For much of the country, however, the change will occur only after the tsunami hits!

 Tsunamis have multiple causes including earthquakes, deep ocean avalanches, and volcanic activity.

Discontent with the American health care system is evident from multiple vantage points.

- Consumers want a less costly system but don't want to ante up more money to support their expensive tastes in health care.
- Business wants maximal cost control with little responsibility.
- The federal government wants a system that is equitable for all American citizens and in which costs are covered by other payers.
- Providers want maximal profit with minimal interference.
- Payers want to be left alone.
- And everyone else is essentially confused by the complexity of health care delivery in the United States.

At the same time, there is a growing consensus that there are multiple underlying issues that will affect the future of health care delivery in our nation. A sampling of the major issues includes:

- Rising costs of health care will require changes in reimbursement mechanisms and policies.
- The role of clinical providers will shift dramatically in response to cost pressures, community needs, and outcomes research.
- The threat of a bankrupt Medicare program will necessitate a major overhaul by Congress.

- Restructuring of the health care system will result in integration of services.
- Health care services will become more customer-focused and personalized.
- New and evolving applications of health technology will be realized if they offer increased productivity or efficiency to the system.

Each of these issues contributes to *The Turnaround Imperative* evident in health care.

 There is a substantial time delay from the creation of a tsunami to when it finally hits shore.

It has taken the past decade for the momentum in health care reform to culminate in serious proposals. The missing element was leadership. The policy deliberations of the Clinton Administration served as a catalyst for change in health care. Leadership from the White House and the Congress together is a requisite—but insufficient—ingredient in the health care reform debate. Even though health care reform failed in 1994, the face of reform will rise again. Why? Because it goes way beyond politics. That's why Newt Gingrich has introduced the new Republican Medicare Plus plan. If it fails, other proposals will follow—until something changes. Political leadership is not creating the health care tsunami, but rather acknowledging the inescapable conclusion that health care reform is crucial for the nation. The lesson of tsunamis is that they cannot be held back. They are inevitable—just like reform of American health care.

 The tsunami is silent and often goes unnoticed until it reaches its destination.

A tsunami is invisible, runs deep, and is silent until it hits shore. At sea, sailors most frequently do not even notice when a tsunami passes by. Why? Because the shore—the destination—is what creates the destruction. Out in the ocean, a wave can dissipate into the depths of the ocean. Close to shore, there is not the ability to dissipate into the depths. As a result, the tsunami becomes an imperative as the wave comes closer to shore.

Because they are not environmentally aware, many institutions that dot the shore line of health care are missing the cues that could alert them to the need to prepare for impending changes in the system. In recent years, much has been written about the need for vision in health care. However, for many health care leaders, their lack of vision has allowed the health care tsunami to reach the shores of many institutions across the nation. The wave has reached its destination and havoc will reign for the next several years. Such is the nature of tsunamis.

The Two Faces of Lituya Bay

Lituya Bay is a picturesque inlet that lies in the Alaskan panhandle, 150 miles north of Sitka. The bay is framed on three sides by majestic cliffs that rise from the ocean. The inlet, although seemingly quiet and calm because it is protected by the cliffs, has long been known as a death trap by the Tlingit Indians. According to legends, the bay is inhabited by a jealous demon who dwells deep in the bay and, when provoked by strangers, thrashes about to splash water on and capture them.

We now know that the cause of the great waves is a large geological fault that lies under the bay. Whenever an earthquake occurs in this area, it causes massive destruction of the cliffs and displacement of the bay floor. All of the floor movement creates massive waves—the largest in the world. On July 9, 1958, a great earthquake shook the bay and unleashed 90 million tons of rock from the cliffs. The rocks came from as high as 3,000 feet and plunged into the bay. The massive fall of rock produced a huge wave that swept from the bay into the ocean. Scientists who later examined the area were astonished to find that the wave had surged to 1,740 feet—the greatest tsunami wave ever recorded.

 Receding water is a signal that a tsunami is on the way.

Decreasing hospital occupancy rates, replacement of traditional indemnity insurance with increased managed care enrollment, an inadequate supply of primary care providers, and reduced growth rates in traditional core services are all signs of an impending tsunami wave in health care. These are all signs that the demand for "business as usual" is decreasing. And, as with the tsunami, once the water begins to recede, it's too late to get to higher ground.

In the hospital industry, a target (of late) for non-Medicare days per thousand has been around 300. Many institutions in aggressive managed care marketplaces are dealing with environments that are pushing 150 days per thousand, and these organizations are planning for less than 100 days per thousand utilization. But if less than 100 days per thousand is feasible, why not consider less than 70 days per thousand by the end of the decade.

The Destruction of Tsunamis

1755: An earthquake rocks the city of Lisbon, Portugal, and, together with a tsunami, destroys the city, killing an estimated 60,000 people.

1783: An earthquake rocks the Calabria region of Italy. A large whirlpool forms and strikes the bay, causing the destruction of the lighthouse. Observers of the time note that deep water fish called cicirelli were found in abundance on the surface of the bay following the whirlpool.

1883: Krakatoa Volcano in the East Indies erupts, and the entire island collapses into the sea with a depth of only 820 feet. A tsunami forms and hits the coasts of Sumatra and Java, killing 36,000 people, with water walls that reach 115 feet in height.

1896: The eastern coast of Japan is battered by a tsunami with waves 80 to 115 feet high. Over 100,000 homes are destroyed, and 26,000 people are killed.

1946: Unimak Island, off the coast of Alaska, is hit by an earthquake that sets off a tsunami. The tsunami hits the Scotch Cap Lighthouse, which is destroyed with five men inside, and the lighthouse is 32 feet above sea level! A radio antennae that is further up the shore at 103 feet is also destroyed. But that isn't all. The tsunami travels to Hawaii—about 2,300 miles away—and hits without warning. Thirty- to 50-foot waves hit Hilo. The tsunami kills 159 people and damages the shoreline.

1964: A great earthquake hits Alaska, causing the formation of a tsunami that spreads across the Pacific Ocean at speeds of up to 400 miles per hour. All along the western coast of the United States, large waves hit the shores causing massive destruction. Fourteen hours after the tremor, the tsunami hits the coast line of Japan in a massive surge—4,000 miles from the source of the tsunami.

1994: A 20-foot wave hits the coast of Indonesia at night after a large earthquake at sea. Thousands are left homeless as a result.

> ***Despite the availability of warning systems,***
> ***the tsunami is very destructive when it finally hits,***
> ***if you don't prepare!***

In areas where the tsunami has a tradition of periodically appearing, communities brace for the devastation through preparation. How? Where there is a history of a tsunami hitting the shore line, communities have learned through the ages to build their infrastructures on higher ground. Schools, central services, hospitals, and other important institutions for sustaining the community are not built on the beaches.

There are multiple warning signs flashing in the debate on health care reform. Virtually every day, a newspaper, magazine, or professional journal contains some analysis of the changes in health care. Despite the admonitions, however, many health care organizations are either unprepared or do not know how to change. Because tsunamis will inevitably hit the health care shores, the end result is *The Turnaround Imperative*.

References

1. Walker, B. *Earthquake*. Alexandria, Va.: Time-Life Books, 1982, p. 26.
2. Vaill, P. *Managing as a Performing Art: New Ideas for a World of Chaotic Change*. San Francisco, Calif.: Jossey-Bass Publishers, 1989.
3. Morgan, G. *Riding the Waves of Change: Developing Managerial Competencies for a Turbulent World*. San Francisco, Calif.: Jossey-Bass Publishers, 1989.
4. Gribbin, J. *This Shaking Earth*. New York, N.Y.: Putnam, 1978, p. 135.

CHAPTER II

What Is a Turnaround?

The Ultimate Change Experience

"If you can dream—and not make dreams your master;
If you can think—and not make thoughts your aim;
If you can meet with Triumph and Disaster
And treat those two impostors just the same..."

Rudyard Kipling
"If"

Surfing the Tsunami

The whole notion of turnaround is new to our lexicon and evolved out of changes in corporate America during the 1980s. Tenneco and IBM are but a few notable examples of corporate turnarounds that have been described extensively in the business literature. Although there is much to learn from the business literature, it seems that there are some peculiarities within the health care industry.

Based on our experience and a review of the few articles and books[1-6] that have been written on the subject, we define a turnaround as "a rapid organizational response involving multiple, simultaneous leadership activities and changes that will dictate the institution's future."

The turnaround involves consideration of the change continuum. The continuum consists of developmental, strategic, and transformational responses[7] (see the table on page 15). Most organizations engage in some type of ongoing, developmental or strategic change. And such activities are usually comfortable and familiar to the organization. In contrast to this, turnaround situations include conditions that force an organization to engage in urgent, simultaneous initiatives resulting in transformational change.

As an example, in the pre-1983, non-DRG, stable, fee-for-service environment, developmental change was an acceptable approach for most health care entities. In the 1980s, a more strategic approach was required. Now that the rapid and often unpredictable changes of the 1990s are upon us, a transformational change response will be required in those organizations that did not adequately prepare for the coming tsunamis.

A developmental change response (figure 1, page 13) is incremental in nature and improves on the present state of things. As a response to change pressures within an organization, the developmental approach is much more prevalent in secure and stable environments, most often occurring while an organization is in a dominant market position. It tends to preserve the status quo through the maintenance of institutional prerogatives, mission, and structure. Because it is not dramatic or threatening, a developmental change response is frequently understood, accepted, and embraced by followers. In predictable and sustainable environments, a developmental change response is a natural process that can occur under management with or without good leadership.

Strategic change responses (figure 2, page 13) move an organization from an old state to a new state that can be articulated over a controlled period; generally, there is no crisis. The magnitude of change can be significant and may involve altered organizational structures and directions. However, the imperative to change may not be as obvious as in a turnaround situation. The strategic change response must be directed by leadership that understands and is either in line with or ahead of outside forces.

FIGURE 1. Developmental Change[7]

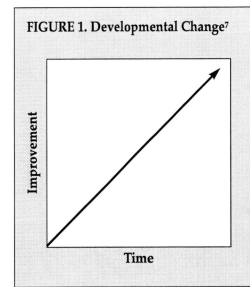

- *Incremental in nature and improves on the present state of the organization. Tends to preserve the status quo.*

- *Health care in the 1970s.*

FIGURE 2. Strategic Change[7]

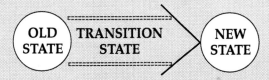

- *Moves the organization from an old state to a new state.*
- *Produces significant change and may involve altered organizational structures and directions.*

- *Health care in the 1980s.*

Good management is one ingredient in a successful strategic change process; leadership is crucial. The result is evolutionary—not revolutionary—change within the organization through a planned, proactive process. Successful strategic organizational change also most frequently involves collaboration with the work force. From an environmental perspective, it is rhythmic and anticipated.

The transformational change response forces (figure 3, page 14) the organization to reemerge after a period of chaos into a new state that is most often not known during the initial phase of the change response. There is nothing like moving in a direction and not knowing exactly where you're going! Instead, where you are going evolves as part of an overall transformational strategy.

Frequently, *The Turnaround Imperative* for an organization is a last ditch effort to save it in a chaotic environment that requires urgent and revolutionary responses, involving power and coercive strategies. Because time is of the essence, the developmental and strategic change responses will not be sufficient. They come later and will ensure completion of the turnaround situation by helping the organization sustain its new direction.

■ **FIGURE 3. Transformational Change[7]**

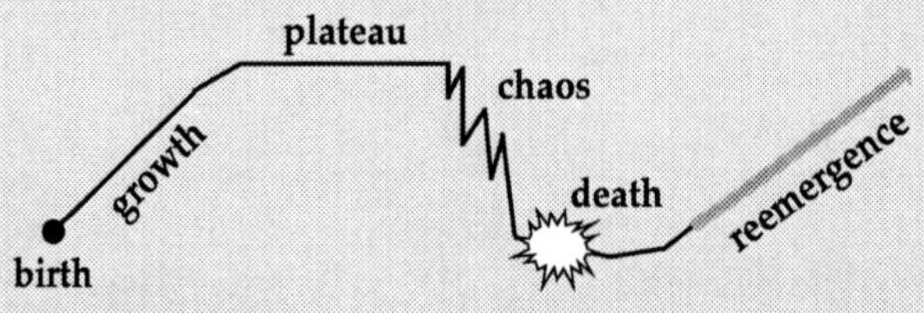

- *Forces the organization to reemerge from a period of chaos into a new state not known during the initial phase of the change process.*

- *Health care in the 1990s and beyond.*

The hospital is the perfect example of how changes can occur within an institution at different times in different environments. In the 1970s, most hospitals operated at capacity, considered expansion of their inpatient capacity, and faced no fiscal problems due to constrained reimbursement. A developmental change strategy was adequate. In the 1980s, with the advent of the Medicare prospective payment system, hospitals began to experience overcapacity, a decline in inpatient utilization, and increasingly severe fiscal problems. Smart institutions with good leaders began to use strategic change responses for adapting the mission of the organization to the new environment. Today, all health care leaders live in a time requiring transformational change responses. Some are burying their heads in the sand and can expect devastating consequences from the coming tsunamis. Others have developed capabilities and mindsets to survive the tsunamis and may emerge stronger.

The Change Continuum: An Analysis of Turnaround Change Responses		
Developmental	**Strategic**	**Transformational**
Health care in the 1970s	Health care in the 1980s	Health care in the 1990s and Beyond
evolutionary	managed	revolutionary
sequential	constructed	simultaneous
logical	strategic	reactive
responsive	compelling	mandatory
incremental	metered	urgent
controlled	planned	chaotic
predictable	anticipated	unpredictable
finite	variable	erratic
leadership understands outside forces	leadership responds to outside forces	leadership anticipates outside forces
procedural	process	power
end state predictable	end state envisioned	end state uncertain
understood	embraced	resisted
slow	measured	dramatic
Smooth Sailing!	Small Craft Warnings!	Tsunami Watch!

Underlying the change continuum are six key principles for turnarounds:

Principle of Simultaneity—A turnaround is not a sequential exercise or series of events. Rather, multiple processes occur concurrently and unpredictably, requiring the mastery of different problems and issues simultaneously by the leader. Leaders who are incapable of dealing with multiple demands originating from different sources and with differing priorities will be thwarted in their efforts to lead a turnaround situation.

Principle of Rapidity—The simultaneous nature of turnaround elements coupled with the accelerated decision making and change required in recreating the organization demands a unique leadership pace. Furthermore, in our experience, the pace cannot be sustained over protracted periods except through extra-human effort.

Principle of Complexity—Complexity evolves from the requirements on the leader to simultaneously manage the old organization while defining a vision for the new entity. In addition, the leader must blend the two entities into a coherent framework for those who are assisting in creating the new order in a chaotic environment.

15

Principle of Uncertainty—Decisions in turnarounds never seem to be black or white. The grey zone dominates turnaround decisions. The leader often is faced with pioneering new concepts for the organization that provide no guarantee of effectiveness for the turnaround effort.

Principle of Management by Intuition—In situations demanding simultaneous, rapid decisions in complex and uncertain situations, there is a high need for intuitive thinking. The ability to see possibilities and patterns with the limited information available and to act on hunches is an important element of effective functioning as a leader in a turnaround situation.

Principle of Leader Objectivity—Impassioned objectivity is an absolute need in the turnaround leader. Without it, the leader will succumb to old relationships, use unreliable information, and remain wedded to existing paradigms of the organization facing a turnaround.

Except for the "Principle of Leader Objectivity," the principles of the turnaround situation are akin to the art of juggling. If you were to decide to juggle, your natural inclination would be to adopt a left-brain strategy by examining the process of juggling. As in most learning, we would read instructions, review charts, and take it in steps.

But juggling—like the turnaround—is a right-brain activity. In right-brain exercises, we let go! We use awareness, mental agility, and creativity to solve problems, not lists and processes. The principles outlined above involve a right-brain approach to problem-solving.

References

1. Goldston, M. *The Turnaround Prescription—Repositioning Troubled Companies.* San Francisco, Calif.: Jossey-Bass Publishers, 1992.

2. Marszalek-Gaucher, E., and Coffey, R. Transforming Healthcare Organizations: How to Achieve and Sustain Organizational Excellence. San Francisco, Calif.: Jossey-Bass Publishers, 1990.

3. Atchison, T. *Turning Health Care Leadership Around—Cultivating Inspired, Empowered and Loyal Followers.* San Francisco, Calif.: Jossey-Bass Publishers, 1990.

4. Silver, A. *The Turnaround Survival Guide: Strategies for the Company in Crisis.* Dearborn, Mich.: Dearborn Financial Publishing, Inc., 1991.

5. Baehr, R. *Engineering a Hospital Turnaround: Proven Strategies for Reinvigorating Financial and Operating Performance.* San Francisco, Calif.: Jossey-Bass Publishers, 1993.

6. Beckhard, R., and Pritchard, W. Changing the Essence: *The Art of Creating and Leading Fundamental Change in Organizations.* San Francisco, Calif.: Jossey-Bass Publishers, 1992.

7. Ackerman, L. "Development, Transition, or Transformation: The Question of Change in Organizations." *OD Practitioner*, Dec. 1986.

CHAPTER III

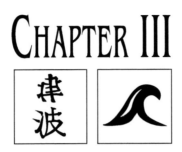

Why Turnarounds?

The Change Imperative in Health Care

"If we do not change our direction, we are very likely to end up exactly where we are headed."

Anonymous

The Tsunami Warning

Change and health care are becoming synonymous concepts—or, as we recently shared with a planning group, health care and change are redundant statements. Multiple drivers in the health system are forcing a reassessment of traditions within in the industry. These drivers are also precipitating the need for a different type of health care leader, one who can anticipate and respond to the changing environmental challenges through new behavior and approaches.

In essence, we are facing a revolution in health care. Noel Tichy, PhD, of the University of Michigan has articulated the issue well: "The U.S. health care system is a striking example of the need for revolution. I still hold out optimism, yet it is far more guarded than in 1986. The 21st Century winners will be those who are in constant revolution. Unfortunately, transformation leaders are in short supply. There are few role models in the world of successful transformations. Revolution calls for leaders with the head, heart, and guts to improve the world. It requires taking on the challenge of creatively destroying and remaking organizations on a continual basis. It is painful. There will be dislocations, people will lose jobs, power will be shifted, hospitals will be closed, people's livelihoods affected. Revolutions are predictable. The pain, the resistance, the breakthroughs, and the joys of successful passage from one phase to another can be understood and mastered."

Environmental Trends in the Health Industry

Everywhere we turn as health care leaders, there is evidence of major change. Reimbursement methodologies are undergoing radical alteration, traditionally stable institutions are being challenged, new organizational models are evolving, the types and roles of providers best suited to provide care are being questioned, and consumer expectations are heightened. The challenge today is understanding the pace of changes in health care for the future.

To understand what the future holds for the health care industry, it is critical to examine and understand major trends that are reinventing the future of health care systems.

 HEALTHTREND: The rising costs of health care will demand changes in payment methodologies.

Aside from the actual dollar amount invested in the United States on health care, the rate of increase in health care expenditures is a major problem. Health care costs are presently doubling every seven years. The American public is increasingly discontented with the costs of health care and is beginning to demand more control of health care costs. Furthermore, the business community is increasingly vocal on the need for curbing the growth of health care costs. We can anticipate that this debate will accelerate in the 1990s.

The Turnaround Imperatives

International comparisons. Per capita health care costs of other nations are appreciably lower than those in the United States, and yet comparable outcomes and similar health status are achieved.

Global economy. Participation in the global economy requires that goods and services produced in the United States be competitive in multiple marketplaces. The marginal contribution of health care costs can be a prohibitive factor in whether or not those goods and services are competitive in foreign markets.

Limited national resources. The national budget is facing continual pressure from multiple societal demands and constituencies in the face of increasingly defined limits. The internal competition for limited resources will force all stakeholders to demonstrate maximal efficiency and productivity.

Provider participation. In an era of constrained resources, those with the best knowledge of the system must participate in decisions on how best to use those resources, and they must be held accountable for those decisions. In health care, providers and managers of the system have not traditionally been held accountable for these areas.

> *HEALTHTREND: The role of clinical providers is shifting dramatically in response to cost pressures, community needs, and outcomes research.*

The physician has been the centerpiece of the health care workforce for decades. As the health care system becomes more sophisticated and it's practitioners become more knowledgeable about how best to delivery all elements of care by matching health problems with the most appropriate resources, pressure will be applied to traditional delivery systems. Although the role of the physician will continue, it will no doubt be less dominant than in prior decades, particularly in primary care because of the evolution of nonphysician providers such as physician assistants and nurse practitioners.

The Turnaround Imperatives

Insufficient numbers of primary care physicians. An inadequate number of primary care physicians has been a problem in our society for the past 20 years. The problem has been exacerbated by a decline in the number of students selecting primary care fields over the past decade. The trend has reversed itself only in the past year. The lack of primary care physicians is creating a substantial opportunity for other health care providers to enter the marketplace with primary care skills.

Outcomes accreditation. The evolving roles of all clinical providers will move the delivery role to the denominator of the cost equation. Maximal services will be demanded from providers at less cost and with an expectation of outcomes of equivalent quality. Rather than measuring competency according to the particular training program completed by a health professional, we could engage in outcomes accreditation based on the demonstrated capabilities of the individual health professional. Such an approach would radically alter the current hierarchy within the health care professions.

 HEALTHTREND: *The fundamental incentives of the health care system are shifting quickly.*

The health care system is driven by incentives and, in some cases, by a lack of incentives. The traditional approach to health care has been driven by volume. For example, if the number of beds is held constant, the hospital occupancy rate for 1980 was 78 percent. In 1992, the occupancy rate would have dropped to 67 percent. In systems where capitated incentives exist, the occupancy rate would have plummeted in a range of 46 percent to a mere 18 percent.[2] No longer is volume the driver of the system.

The Turnaround Imperatives

Managed care. Increasing domination of the health care system by managed care and capitated payment systems will shift incentives toward different modalities of delivery that are more cost efficient. Efficiency, productivity, and preventive strategies are the hallmarks of the new health care system. The primary focus will be not on maximization of reimbursement but on cost-effective use of limited resources. Markets such as Minneapolis, Minnesota; Madison, Wisconsin; Seattle, Washington; San Francisco, California; and others are experiencing rapid growth in managed care activity. For example, prepaid programs represent about 65 percent of payments to physicians in the San Francisco area.

Geographic focus. Health care will be delivered geographically in defined regions. Incentives under such a system are driven by community needs as defined by the population in the geographic area.

Preventive focus. Pressure will mount to move health services *upstream* toward preventive services. In fact, capitation of the system can allow creative approaches by health care providers in emphasizing prevention as a mainstay of primary care.

 HEALTHTREND: *Restructuring of the health care system will result in integration of services*

Clear trends of collaboration between providers and purchasers of health care are beginning to occur. Further alignment of hospitals, physicians, and insurance carriers, including health maintenance organizations and preferred provider organizations, into consolidated and possibly closed systems will evolve. Many health care futurists are predicting total integration of traditionally separate turfs within the health care environment. Specifically, groups of physicians will become integrated with hospitals. The development of regional health care systems requires this close integration of services and coordination of service delivery, especially as the system moves toward prepaid health care systems, which is projected to be the dominant force in health care finance by the end of the 1990s.

🏄 The Turnaround Imperatives

Multispecialty practice. Increased dominance of health care by multispecialty groups will become the norm. By 1988, the number of group practices had grown to more than 16,500 and employed more than 155,600 physicians. Between 1965 and 1988, an estimated 448 percent increase in the number of physicians in groups occurred.[3] By 1990, one of every three physicians was part of a group, with at least 50 percent of those physicians in multispecialty practices. It is estimated that more than 50 percent of all practicing physicians in the United States are now in group situations.

Alternative practice patterns. All providers will receive fixed incomes as their financial base in the future. Related to the group phenomenon are the increasing numbers of part-time equivalent physicians engaged in practices. Although not exclusively a result of increased numbers of women physicians, data support the notion that women are much more frequently inclined to engage in part-time practices. Women presently represent about 40 percent of the entering medical school classes across the nation. Increased emphasis on less-than-full-time practices is evident among male physicians, as well. Any discussion with medical students would quickly reveal the importance of *lifestyle* as a valuable commodity in selecting a specialty. The growth of emergency medicine is a good example of physicians engaging in a fixed-income specialty with a designated number of hours. Once again, an environment that allows such practice patterns (e.g., group practice or hospital-based practice) is clearly the desired option of these providers.

Ambulatory focus. Accelerated movement of health services toward ambulatory settings will occur. It is projected by some analysts that, by the close of the 1990s, 90 percent of diagnostic work and 70 percent of therapeutic work will be conducted in the outpatient setting. Leland Kaiser, PhD., a noted health care futurist, predicts that, by 2000:

- Acute care will consume only 30 percent of the nation's health care budget (i.e., $450 billion, equivalent to total 1986 health care expenditures).
- Ambulatory care will consume 45 percent of the budget (i.e., $675 billion, equivalent to 1990 national health care expenditures).
- Home care will represent 25 percent of the health care dollar (i.e., $375 billion).

Furthermore, it is anticipated that, by 2000, 20 percent of existing acute care beds will not exist. Such rapid moves toward a different modality of health care delivery will result in stress in the system. Preparing for such changes would seem an advisable strategy.

Corporatization of health care. In recent years, the health care industry has seen a marked increase in the number of corporate entities providing services. The health care environment has moved from a "mom and pop," local, isolated operation into an organized, regional, and even national scope that integrates the full spectrum of health care services. The projection of most analysts in the health industry is for the trend to continue.

Collaborative and cooperative health care networks. Many health care consultants note the development of regional networks for hospitals, long-term care programs, physician practices, and the like. Massive consolidation is beginning to occur in selected geographic areas. For example, in Milwaukee, Wisconsin, health care is becoming a totally integrated activity dominated by three major institutions. Such consolidation is anticipated in much of the nation.

Provider executives and leaders. Management of health systems will move toward the addition of senior managers who have a foundation in clinical training as well as strong administrative skills. The coupling of traditional health care leaders with strong clinical executives will create a dynamic synergy in organizational strength that can meet the challenges of the new health care system.

Governance. Real power and decision making must be shared in the future between traditional administrators, boards of directors, and physician leaders to facilitate effective participation of clinicians in resource allocation decisions. The token clinician representative in governance is over. Structures must be modified to accomplish this important objective.

 HEALTHTREND: Health care services will become more customer-focused and personalized.

The total quality movement in health care will not diminish. The health care system, although later than most industries, now realizes the importance of customer input and satisfaction. Health care institutions have made major strides in reengineering and refining their processes to become more customer-sensitive. These processes have resulted in an increased sensitivity to the types of programs and services required of health care organizations.

The Turnaround Imperatives

Types of services. Altered pressures on the types of services needed from the health care setting will begin to occur. Much consideration has been given to the increased numbers of elderly who will require care in future decades. The increase in the demand for services by the elderly will cause strain on the system, especially if the national economic situation does not improve relative to the global economy. Other chronic problems, such as AIDS, the secondary effects of crack cocaine usage on children, and other societal maladies will also have an impact on the health care system.

Outcomes management. Both clinical and educational components of health care will become more outcomes focused in the late 1990s. As part of the continuous quality improvement movement in health care and other industries, we are seeing more emphasis on the "outcomes" of particular strategies or interventions. Management of outcomes has become the major emphasis of the health care industry in recent years and will no doubt continue.

 HEALTHTREND: *New and evolving applications of health technology.*

The use of technology will radically alter our whole concept of health care over the course of the next decade. We are on the threshold of breakthrough technological applications similar to the introduction of sterile technique in surgery and the use of antibiotics in medicine.

Technology applications. Technology is already rapidly altering the health care environment. The introduction of laparoscopic surgery has radically changed the approach to such problems as gallbladder surgery. Over a period of a few short years, the traditional cholecystectomy admission moved from a hospital-based procedure that resulted in a six- to nine-inch scar with an average three- to seven-day length of stay at a cost of $7,000 to $10,000 to an ambulatory procedure leaving a tiny scar on the abdomen with a stay of less than 24 hours at a cost of $4,000 to $5,000. In looking to the future, laparoscopic surgery may soon become obsolete for certain procedures.

Biotechnology. In looking back on health care in the 1990s, historians will note the impact of the Human Genome Project on health care. In fact, the project may be one of the lasting legacies of our generation for centuries to come. We are now at the forefront of emerging technologies that will allow us to affect the health of an individual at the cellular level. The changes that will result are, for the moment, incomprehensible and pose numerous ethical complexities.

Telecommunications. The computer is the provider's next stethoscope! Not only will the information highway allow for the transfer of information at regional and national levels, but also processing within the institution will become ever more sophisticated as the computer becomes an adjunct tool in the delivery of health care.

References

1. Tichy, N. "The Three-Act Revolutionary Drama." *Healthcare Forum Journal* 36(4):51-5, July-Aug. 1993.
2. The Governance Committee. *Capitation Strategy.* Washington, D.C.: The Advisory Board, 1994, p. 11.
3. Havlicek, P. *Medical Groups in the United States.* Chicago, Ill.: American Medical Association, 1990, pp. 33-9.

CHAPTER IV

The Organizational Assessment

Evaluating the Turnaround Situation

"In the long run, most men hit what they aim at."

Henry David Thoreau

High Tide versus a Tsunami

Health care leaders will inevitably be faced with potential turnaround situations during the coming decade. Chapter II developed a description and definition of a turnaround situation. In considering the challenge of leading a turnaround, a series of organizational questions must be asked by the leader. The answers to these questions will determine the magnitude of the turnaround situation and the leader's potential for success.

Turnaround Considerations

Now that we've defined the global issues in a turnaround, it is important to define the other major organizational issues that contribute to why turnarounds occur? There are any number of specific reasons for a turnaround situation, and there is no cookie-cutter set of reasons. At the same time, there is a set of considerations that seem to apply to all turnaround situations and that fall into three broad categories: business and finance, leadership and human resources, and organizational culture. Each consideration individually contributes to the overall environment of a turnaround. Although each consideration may precipitate a turnaround situation, the norm is that more than one reason exists. Also, a multiplier effect exists, whereby recognition of additional considerations accentuates the probability of a turnaround situation. In other words, the more elements that are evident in an organization, the greater the likelihood that a turnaround will eventually be required.

 Consideration One: Business and Finance

■ Unrecognized Decline in the Core Business.

A turnaround is on the horizon when investments continue to be made in the core business areas in the face of ongoing market share losses. One of the best examples of a failure to recognize a decline in the core business is the decision by an acute care facility to invest substantial funds in a *plant replacement project* to replicate the historical functions. Is this the future of health care in America?

Questions:

❚ What complement of services did the organization provide at its zenith?

❚ Which core services have declined or have been eliminated in the past two years? Why?

❚ How have market demographics changed in the past two years?

❚ Has the service area of the organization declined?

❚ Are the current core services and programs oriented toward the future?

❚ What is the status of the organization with accreditation bodies?

❚ What is the reputation of the organization among peers?

❚ Why should this organization survive?

■ Cash Flow a Continuous Problem.

Cash flow is one of the key indicators of a potential turnaround situation. Frequently, there is concern over meeting payroll and paying bills in a timely manner. In the face of such a dilemma, even aggressive accounts receivable management does not eliminate the cash flow problem for the organization. Management is either unwilling or incapable of taking corrective actions to manage the cash flow situation. Because the values of the health care industry involve helping people, serious discussions about downsizing or reengineering within the organization are often more difficult than in other more financially driven industries. In reality, cash flow cannot be managed in health care without attention to these areas because of the heavy dependence on human resources for delivering the product and services called health care.

Small rural hospitals, when faced with declining inpatient census and inflated staffing ratios, have too frequently engaged in across-the-board unpaid time off rather than focusing decisions on whether or not a wing of the institution should be closed. How will a strategy that marginally affects all employees generate sufficient cash to support a failing unit?

Questions:

▮ What is the organization's payer mix?

▮ What is the penetration of managed care? Of capitated products?

▮ Are pricing strategies current?

▮ Do financial ratios reveal the origin of financial problems?

▮ To what degree are reserves being used to offset cash flow problems?

■ Research and Development Investments and Initiatives Are Marginal.

Research and development investments, *a priori*, involve risk. Too frequently, the first cuts for the organization facing a turnaround situation are in the R&D area. Such an approach is strong evidence of a lack of strategic focus within the organization. Furthermore, mechanisms are not in place to allow the organization to pursue the development of innovative products or initiatives. As a result, organizational leadership continues to believe it must use its limited resources to protect what is currently in place rather than to develop what must be.

A health care organization that fails to invest sufficient resources in the development of clinical outcome parameters will continue to have ineffective tools for managing quality and resource allocation. Is the best investment in traditional quality assurance methodologies or in the development of data systems to support clinical continuous quality improvement initiatives?

Questions:

▮ What percentage of overall expenditures are allocated to research and development initiatives?

▮ What new programs are supported through internal funds?

▮ Have outside funds been generated to support new program development?

∎ Are internal processes in place to stimulate innovative thinking?

∎ What R & D efforts is the organization proud of?

■ Planning Is Rote, *not* Dynamic.

We are convinced that many organizations simply do not have a clear sense of planning as a change-oriented process. The planning model within the organization is dominated by *micro thinking* (inside out), which results in preparation of documents that focus on maintaining the status quo. In a turnaround situation, however, it is imperative that the organization step back and engage in a *macro thinking* (outside in) process, which reconsiders basic business assumptions and strategies of the organization.

Health care organizations often treat their planning process as an endless compilation of objectives and action plans—a hopelessly insufficient activity! For what changes are these committed individuals preparing the plans?

Questions:

∎ Does the organization offer any unique services to the community or region? Are those services still needed?

∎ If you could start the business over again, what would be the core services?

∎ What are competitors doing?

∎ Has an environmental scan been conducted in the past year? What were the results?

∎ Does the strategic planning process involve all levels of the organization, especially the CEO and senior management team?

■ Capital Investments Lack Future Thinking.

Too frequently, capital investments that precipitated a turnaround situation revolved around the needs and prerogatives of managers rather than the needs and prerogatives of the organization. In fact, for many turnaround situations, the key investments that are required often involve areas in which there is insufficient leadership. Traditional investments geared toward sustaining the past rather than carrying the organization forward are frequently a major underlying cause of many turnaround situations.

In the health care industry, we frequently make investment decisions on the basis of the wants and needs of a few physicians in power positions (e.g., high admitters, leaders on the medical staff). Should the progressive health care system invest huge amounts of capital in a new cardiac catheterization lab for the cardiologists or in management information systems to support its future in an industry that is quickly becoming information-dependent?

Questions:

∎ To what degree have capital assets deteriorated over the past two years?

∎ What are the major *perceived* capital needs of the organization?

∎ What are the major *real* capital needs of the organization?

■ What have been the historical investments by the organization in its infrastructure over the past three years?

Consideration Two: Leadership and Human Resources

■ Leadership Is Status Quo-Oriented and Lacks Energy and Determination.

Organizational change—especially transformational change—requires an incredible amount of energy and determination on the part of leadership. Leaders who have been in the organization for a long time are frequently quite comfortable with the status quo. They see changes as threatening to their position and status within the organization. With such leaders, there is a lack of impetus to engage in any type of meaningful change effort. The result is an organization that, over time, suffers from insufficient leadership investment—a problem that can be as deadly as insufficient capital investments.

Characteristic of many academic medical centers are physician educators and leaders whose purpose is concentrated on maintaining the status, size, and personal interests associated with members of their departments. Does anyone doubt the need for academic medical centers to develop a more integrated strategy in order to sustain their very important role in health care for society?

Questions:

■ How long has leadership been in its current position?

■ Was leadership recently changed? If so, what for? If not, why?

■ What is the leader's vision of the future for the organization?

■ Has leadership admitted its responsibility for or contribution to the current organizational problems?

■ Is there a management team whose members work together in a cohesive fashion?

■ Do members of the management team feel comfortable in challenging one another about the organization's future?

■ Is the CEO clear about the important future decisions that will need to be made and is he or she willing to make them?

■ Blame Is Continuously Shifted Away from Leadership.

Key responsibilities for change within an organization reside at the leadership level—with the board, upper management, and departmental levels. The important thing to remember about leadership within organizations is that people "below" take their cues from those who are "above." In potential turnaround situations, leadership has frequently been successful in transferring blame to other levels of the organization.

Hard decisions are often left to management by a caretaker board of directors that is disengaged from the problems of the organization. How many organizations in crisis do you know where bottom-up leadership can be effective in sustaining major change?

Questions:

▮ Is there fear among managers of being blamed for problems?

▮ What are the incentive systems of the organization?

▮ When was the last employee survey conducted?

▮ Are there data regarding employee morale?

▮ Does the organization engage in a regular chief executive officer evaluation?

■ Key Staff Members Are Leaving the Organization.

One of the most significant indicators of potential long-range trouble for an organization is the departure of excellent staff members in key positions. Their departure is a signal of underlying problems and a sign that a turnaround is rapidly approaching. Stable staff in the face of a potential turnaround situation could imply either marginal capability among key executives or collusion with the leadership to maintain the status quo. In some cases, excellent staff stay with the organization, despite the mounting evidence of major problems, because of personal considerations, a commitment to the organization, or a recognition of the organization's potential under good leadership.

One area to consider in health care organizations, particularly those that are market driven, is the marketing department. Individuals in these departments are often way ahead of the curve in terms of understanding the market's perception of the organization.

Questions:

▮ Have key managers recently left?

▮ Is there a sense of hopelessness among key managers of the organization?

▮ What types of support systems exist to encourage employees to engage in long-term career planning within the organization?

▮ What is the perspective of human resources on the state of the organization?

▮ What are the major exit interview themes of staff over the past year?

▮ In which key areas of the organization has rapid turnover occurred in recent months?

■ Responsibility for Change Is Assigned with No Authority.

No effective change response can be implemented without real authority, backed up by the commitment of the organization's leadership. Too frequently, leaders espouse the need for change and then delegate the complex change response to staff who are not empowered to implement needed change.

An excellent example of the responsibility-without-authority phenomenon in health care is the lack of success in many continuous quality improvement (CQI) initiatives in the industry. CQI, of necessity, implies changing the basic decision-making process for the organization. In a dysfunctional situation, implementation of a CQI program is assigned to a staff director, while, in reality, the leaders of the organization expect their authority to go unchallenged. Can meaningful change occur without the commitment and involvement of those with control over operational and human resources?

Questions:

▮ What is the organizational structure?

▮ Are reporting relationships among managers clear?

▮ Is a CQI program in place? Is it working?

▮ Can you "walk the talk?"

▮ What is your delegation style?

 Consideration Three: Organizational Culture

■ An Overladen Bureaucracy Stifles Entrepreneurial Energy.

The emphasis of the organization is on maintaining the existing structure and policy rather than on creating opportunities for innovation. The checks and balances of the organization create a culture in which entrepreneurial efforts are met with resistance at every step. A frequent comment to be heard in such an organization is: "That's the way we've always done it!" Such comments are a sign that staff members are ill-prepared for challenges such as tsunami waves.

The home health industry has generally been an enterprise separate from acute and chronic care. In a capitated environment, does it make sense for programs to continue on an independent basis, or should greater programmatic and managerial integration occur?

Questions:

▮ What is the organizational culture?

▮ How are things done in the organization?

▮ What types of policies, procedures, and guidelines are in place?

▮ Can members of the organization articulate its values?

▮ What is the ratio of administrative personnel to staff involved in actual delivery of services or product development?

■ Organizational Culture Does Not Encourage Risk-Taking, Criticism, and Feedback.

Submissive behavior is the norm in a potential turnaround situation. It is not encouraged, but it has, over time, become the organizational norm. Samuel Goldwyn of Metro-Goldwyn-Mayer fame exemplifies the type of culture evident in such organizations when he stated: "I don't want any yes-men around here. I want everyone to tell me the truth even it if costs him his job."[1] In a static culture, other norms begin to develop that hold the organization hostage to meaningful change. Examples include the lack of feedback about leadership behavior, risk-taking behavior on behalf of the organization, and self-criticism as an appropriate internal response to problems of the organization. One of the results of such a culture is that mediocrity is accepted as a norm throughout the organization.

Many independent physician practices operate on an individualistic, command-and-control mentality, which intimidates staff, who, in turn, don't make needed changes in practice. Will it be possible with such a mentality to maintain marketplace position, given the evolution of integrated health care systems?

Questions:

∎ Which ventures failed in the past year and why?

∎ Who talks to the CEO in the lunchroom?

∎ What policies are in place to encourage risk-taking, criticism, and feedback?

∎ Are the organization's values about such behaviors explicit?

∎ Does the organization hold meetings that allow an interchange between staff and leadership?

∎ Covert Behaviors Undermine Formal Organizational Structures.

In organizations that support the cultural norms mentioned above, covert behaviors begin to emerge. They can often be more influential than formal organizational structures in dictating how problems are addressed or resolved. When this occurs, the complexity of internal organizational change is magnified because of the dual systems that must be managed in order to effect needed change.

Some physicians will demonstrate a public commitment to various changes within the health care system and yet engage in private behavior that undermines the organization. Are passive-aggressive behaviors the type of foundation upon which to build a collaborative health care system?

Questions:

∎ Are staff and key constituents affected by the turnaround known for their direct and honest communication?

∎ Are inherent leaders in the organization a part of your communication circle?

∎ Can you share your message directly with everyone in the organization?

∎ Who needs to be watched?

∎ What is your response to behaviors that undermine the turnaround effort?

Conclusion

The result of these turnaround considerations is that change is suppressed, not encouraged, within the organization. Over time in an environment that demands change, the organization will succumb to the need for increasingly transformational responses to ensure success. If organizational leaders are cognizant of the change responses needed, recognize the type of action required, and act accordingly, the turnaround situation may be averted.

Reference

1. Goodman, S. *How to Manage a Turnaround—A Senior Manager's Guide.* New York, N.Y.: Free Press, 1982, p. 26.

CHAPTER V

The Personal Assessment

Why Me, Oh Lord?

"Leaders take us from where we are to where we've never been."

Henry Kissinger

Preventing Wipeout on a Tsunami

The changes sweeping the health care industry will overwhelm many traditional leaders as organizations respond to *The Turnaround Imperative* in the 1990s and beyond. Turnaround situations offer formidable challenges to health care leadership, because the industry has not been previously challenged by such an unstable environment.

The competencies and styles required of the turnaround leader are often foreign to most health care leaders. Why? Because the environment has not demanded their development! The status quo era of the 1970s provided little on-the-job training for health care executives that could enhance their competence as effective change agents. In essence, the major leadership challenge for health care education programs during the coming decade will be in preparing health care executives for a whole new approach to problem solving and management.

There are two definitive stages in a turnaround that demand different leadership styles. The *formative stage,* which occurs in the period immediately following a tsunami and early in the turnaround, is characterized by chaos, confusion, devastation to existing systems and relationships, and the need for immediate action. The leadership style that predominates in the formative stage is authoritarian in nature. The *stabilization stage,* where a vision, mission, and values have been clearly articulated and substantial rebuilding has occurred, is characterized by a more metered approach, clearer direction, a belief in its own survival on the part of the organization, and a renewed optimism about the future. The leadership style that predominates in the stabilization stage is more collaborative in nature.

The turnaround leader must also actively use the six turnaround principles (i.e., simultaneity, rapidity, complexity, uncertainty, management by intuition, and leader objectivity) in decisions. The turnaround leader's inability to utilize these principles as an operational focus will make the turnaround an even more difficult process.

Turnaround leaders must manage the chaos inherent in turnaround situations. Margaret Wheatley, EdD, has written extensively on the topic of chaos management.[1] Her basic premise is that chaos management requires thinking of organizations as complex, living entities rather than as fixed machines with rigid structures. These ideas evolved from the theories of Ilya Prigogine, PhD,[2] who theorized that chaos is the process by which living systems constantly recreate themselves in their environment. Health care organizations are essentially living systems that must engage in re-creation to survive.

When confronted with radical change (i.e., when hit by a tsunami), many of these organizations will simply fall apart. The turnaround leader's challenge is to help the organization redevelop and adapt to the new environment by orchestrating a transformational change response. Turnarounds require confronting and generating energy from chaos.

As the turnaround leader enters the formative stage of the turnaround, the following considerations should be kept in mind.

■ **The leader is often a solo force in determining direction.** The leader must recognize the input of other members of the senior management team and of the workforce. At the same time, turnarounds require immediate leadership action, which often does not allow time to gather input from all sources within the organization. Someone, the turnaround leader, must be willing to make tough decisions in the heat of battle.

■ **The leader must be ready and willing to act.** Because of the speed of change in the turnaround situation, leadership in the formative stage requires a willingness to act on little information. The basis for acting on the part of the turnaround leader is often vision-driven rather than information-driven. William Gates, the President/CEO of Microsoft, articulated the requirements of such leaders when he stated: "In the next couple of years, I will either do the right things or the wrong things to play a role in digital convergence [of computers, phones, and consumer electronics]. People won't really know, they won't be able to recognize whether I did the right things or the wrong things for about five years. But now is the time.[3]

■ **Personal sacrifice is required by the leader.** The demands of the turnaround situation are formidable. Time is short. Resources are frequently scare and poorly organized. All decisions require personal attention rather than delegatory attention. Because the turnaround leader is at the center of all activity involved in the effort, no one seemingly has more information on the gestalt of the turnaround situation than the turnaround leader. The result? Without adequate support systems and personal sustenance, the turnaround leader can become overwhelmed.

■ **The leader must assume a high profile.** In turnaround situations, both internal and external stakeholders want and need access to the leader. Frequent meetings, social encounters, presentations, interactions with media, and other high-profile events are the norm. Whether the leader is an extrovert who thrives on external interactions or an introvert who demands personal reflective space and time, the turnaround requires a very public presence on his or her part.

■ **An ability to force progress with or without consensus is essential.** Visible progress in the early stages of a turnaround is critical to its eventual success. The turnaround leader must find and cultivate successes or victories that demonstrate to everyone that the turnaround is progressing. Although consensus decision-making is an important element in the organization even in the early stages of a turnaround, the leader often does not have time for the consensus process. Staff must clearly understand the implications of such a leadership style. Cohesiveness of the team is important. Empowerment of the team comes later.

Most programs in health and medical management have traditionally concentrated their curricula on the transference of knowledge and skills related to the basics. Although a strong understanding of these areas is absolutely crucial for an effective leader, it is insufficient for the successful turnaround leader in an era of tsunami waves! There is a set of attributes beyond the basics that are becoming increasingly important for health care leaders. Each attribute, including the knowledge and skills required, is discussed below.

Personal Assessment for the Potential Turnaround Leader

For each attribute on the following pages, indicate those knowledge and skill areas you consider to be strengths, weaknesses, or areas in which you need more information.

Attribute: The Basics

Knowledge	*Skills*
An exceptional knowledge and awareness of the health care industry is required. In addition, a recognition must be evident that certain content areas serve as the foundation for all effective leaders. Without a strong understanding and background in these basic areas, the ability to manage change is compromised.	▮ Financial planning and management ▮ Strategic planning ▮ Marketing and public relations ▮ Fund-raising skills ▮ Data analysis ▮ Interpersonal management expertise ▮ Principles of insurance ▮ Computer literacy ▮ Administrative competencies

Personal Self-Assessment:

_____

_____

_____

_____

_____

_____

Attribute: A Facilitative Mentality and Process Orientation

Knowledge	*Skills*
Solid knowledge and understanding of group process are essential elements of a good facilitator. Furthermore, an understanding of quality improvement, the value of data, and reengineering processes is crucial.	▮ Listening ▮ Ability to remain objective and stay out of content ▮ Conflict management ▮ Consensus development ▮ Ability to manage difficult people ▮ Meeting management skills ▮ Ability to develop leadership and cultivate people ▮ Capacity to organize complex, chaotic information

Personal Self-Assessment:

_____

_____

_____

_____

_____

_____

_____

_____

_____

_____

_____

Attribute: A Learning Philosophy

Knowledge	Skills
Recognition that education extends beyond the internal organization to include broad elements of the community outside the traditional realm of health care. Education remains a life-long process for the effective turnaround leader.	▮ Public speaking ▮ Communication—both written and verbal ▮ Constituency building ▮ Ability to learn and profit from mistakes within organizations ▮ Ability to learn lessons from other industries

Personal Self-Assessment:

_____

_____

_____

_____

_____

_____

_____

_____

_____

_____

_____

_____

_____

_____

Attribute: A Sense of Self-Awareness and a Strong Understanding of Personal Strengths and Weaknesses

Knowledge	*Skills*
The self aware leader with a strong sense of personal strengths and weaknesses is important. In particular, an understanding of personal values, standards and choices, and aspirations is crucial for the leader who intends to pursue collaborative strategies or ventures. These attributes must be considered against the backdrop of one's personal vision in order to truly serve as a guide.	▮ Political sensitivity ▮ Understanding of compromise ▮ Awareness of negotiation style ▮ Ability to not let one's ego intervene in the process of developing collaborative strategies or ventures ▮ Ability to admit mistakes and be open to constructive feedback

Personal Self-Assessment:

_____

_____

_____

_____

_____

_____

_____

_____

_____

_____

Attribute: An Awareness of Personal Style and Timing

Knowledge	*Skills*
Timing is highly situational and intuitive. Furthermore, situations usually require different styles and approaches, based on the dynamics of the involved parties. Effective leaders must understand their personal interactive styles to be effective.	▌ Time management ▌ Ability to read other people's leadership styles ▌ Ability to continually monitor situations to clarify the timing of leadership response ▌ Effective communication and listening skills ▌ Ability to give and receive feedback ▌ Flexibility in adapting to a changing environment

Personal Self-Assessment:

_____

_____

_____

_____

_____

_____

_____

_____

_____

_____

_____

Attribute: A Global Perspective

Knowledge	*Skills*
An understanding of broad social, economic, and institutional trends is crucial in assisting the leader to develop health care systems with a meaningful purpose. Lack of knowledge on these trends isolates the leader from the realities of his or her environment.	∎ Ability to articulate a vision ∎ Ability to access, interpret, and manage information ∎ Networking ∎ An understanding of the need to expand boundaries and thinking ∎ Ability to recognize new program and organizational responses to old problems ∎ Community diagnostic skills concerning health issues ∎ Systems thinking and integration ∎ Ability to interpret global trends

Personal Self-Assessment:

_____

_____

_____

_____

_____

_____

_____

_____

_____

_____

_____

41

Attribute: A Team Orientation

Knowledge	Skills
A strong knowledge of team functioning and team building processes. A belief in the potential of teams to contribute to the resolution of complex organizational problems is essential.	▮ Group process techniques ▮ Application of group dynamics ▮ Ability to lead or participate in team initiatives, depending on the needs of the organization ▮ Problem-solving skills ▮ Ability to balance individual and team accountability needs

Personal Self-Assessment:

_____

_____

_____

_____

_____

_____

_____

_____

_____

_____

_____

_____

_____

Conclusion

The Turnaround Imperative will revolutionize management thinking in health care during the coming decade. Traditional skills, while important, will serve only as a foundation for the health care leader of the future. Trends in health care require an evolution in management education provided to leaders, who must be open to understanding new roles for themselves as change agents within health care organizations.

Based on our experience, there is a list of key questions that leaders must ask themselves in a turnaround situation. These questions should be pondered, internally debated, discussed with close friends and colleagues, and openly evaluated with significant others.

- What is my vision for the organization?
- Can I tolerate the ambiguity of simultaneous, rapid change and protect those parts of the organization that require stability?
- Where is the organization in relation to the change continuum?
- How real is the commitment by the organization's leadership (governance) to the resources, changes, and chief executive latitude necessary to be successful?
- Is my leadership style capable of directing a turnaround effort?
- Does my contract provide me with an adequate safety net to take needed risks?
- Who supports change?
- Who resists change?
- What talents exist within the current organization?
- Is there sufficient leader potential in the organization that can be mobilized to assist me in the change effort?
- What personal and professional support systems are in place for me? How can they be developed if they are missing?
- How thick is my skin?
- Can I manage multiple, conflicting perceptions of my style and effectiveness?
- Who can I use as an organizational development or process consultant?
- Am I willing to leave after the turnaround effort is completed, if my skills no longer match the organization's leadership needs?
- Why me?
- Why not?

References

1. Wheatley, M. *Leadership and the New Science: Learning about Organization from an Orderly Universe.* San Francsico, Calif.:Berrett-Koehler, 1993.
2. Prigogine, I., and Stengers, I. *Order Out of Chaos.* New York, N.Y.: Bantam Books, 1984.
3. Interview with Evan Ramstad of the Associated Press, May 1993.

CHAPTER VI

The Turnaround Model:

Putting It All In Perspective

"When your horse dies, dismount."

Richard Warren
Superintendent
Marshfield, Wisconsin, Public School System

Surveying the Damage

Most leaders are ill-equipped to carry forward a successful turnaround. The requirements include training in group facilitation, team development, environmental scanning, forecasting, interviewing, and organizational culture assessment. Furthermore, in the past, the concept of initiating a turnaround in health

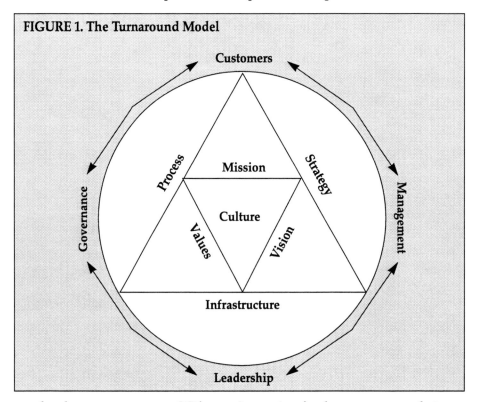

FIGURE 1. The Turnaround Model

care has been an oxymoron. With ever-increasing funds, resources, and strong public support, few turnarounds were precipitated. As a result, not only have management programs neglected to include didactic training, but few health administrators have had experience in the turnaround process.

The overall model used in *The Turnaround Imperative* includes four critical stakeholders—customers, governance, leadership, and management that provide the framework for considering two interrelated triads that serve as the basis for the turnaround model: the operational triad and the philosophical triad. Taken together, these triads contain six components (infrastructure, process, strategy, mission, vision, and values) representing separate functions that occur as part of the turnaround. At the core of these two triads is the organizational culture.

The Operational Triad

Infrastructure. Any turnaround effort requires consideration of infrastructure, which includes space, equipment, information and information systems, agreements and contracts, human resources, structure, and finances. Any turnaround that fails to address each of these areas will not succeed, even with grand strategies and excellent processes.

Strategy. Two types of strategy are inherent in the turnaround. The first strategy element is internally focused and involves activities applied by the leader to the management of the turnaround, such as identifying critical players, building team capacity, and assessing the organization's situation. The second strategy is externally focused and involves development of new strategic directions concerning the organization's future, such as defining new markets and articulating new programs and services (see Chapter IX for a detailed discussion of the topic). Both internal and external elements of strategy are necessary for the successful turnaround.

Process. How the turnaround is accomplished is as much an issue as is what is accomplished. Too frequently, turnaround efforts do not adequately consider process, which includes attention to group dynamics, meeting flow, covert and overt resistance, interpersonal behaviors, styles of interaction, and other organizational dynamics. For example, attendees and meeting agenda and process at the initial retreat that is held to clarify vision and mission can often dictate future success or failure of the turnaround effort. While lack of attention to process may

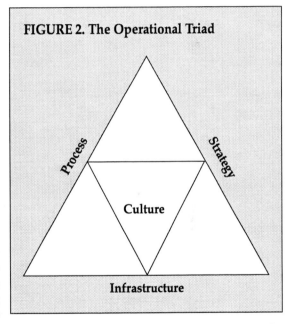

FIGURE 2. The Operational Triad

not be critical in the short-run, it is the undoing of turnaround momentum. The hallmark of truly successful turnaround efforts is creation of sustainable momentum. As a result, attention to the question of process is as critical a function in the formative stage as other elements outlined in this book.

The Philosophical Triad

Vision. There are two dimensions in the successful vision for a turnaround situation. The first involves the vision of the leader, which must be clear and compelling. Without a clear and compelling vision, neither the leader nor the organization can be sustained over time. The second dimension involves buy-in and investment by the four critical stakeholders and others who are important (e.g., employees and regulatory and accreditation bodies) in the turnaround. An inspired vision without the reality of involvement and commitment is just another good idea. Creating the reality out of the rhetoric is the art of the turnaround.

Mission. The mission is basically a description of the here and now situation for the organization. For most organizations, it is the foundation of their work. In a turnaround situation, we find the mission is often out-dated and of little value in inspiring needed change. For this reason, greater emphasis should be placed on the vision statement. However, a clear mission statement must be part of the turnaround effort, because it provides a contrasting framework for evaluating progress toward the vision.

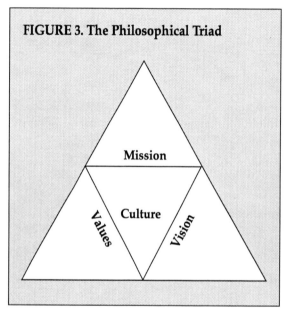

FIGURE 3. The Philosophical Triad

Values. Too little attention is paid to defining and understanding the values of organizations. Yet, inherent values often dictate organizational responses to problems, especially in periods of crisis. The turnaround most frequently requires a reassessment and realignment of organizational values. If values are not clarified, the ability to obtain the personal involvement and commitment required for supporting the turnaround is diminished.

These six components contained in the operational and philosophical triads surround a core area, the organizational culture (see Chapter X). An integrated approach that considers all six components is absolutely necessary. Concentrating energy on any one area to the exclusion of others will undermine the turnaround effort through implementation of an incomplete corporate culture.

The Critical Stakeholder Framework

As noted previously, the framework for each of the six components must be viewed from the four perspectives of the critical stakeholders: customers, governance, leadership, and management. Although there are similarities in the vantage points of these four stakeholders in the turnaround, each has a different role, responsibility, and accountability.

Customers. Customers are the ultimate recipients of products and services for any enterprise. Until recently, the customer did not receive much attention from the health care industry. As competition and change have entered the health care lexicon, however, the focus has shifted dramatically toward the needs of the customer.

The ultimate customer in health care is the individual patient. Other customers include payers, providers, communities, and other external stakeholders. The reactions of customers and their stakes in the turnaround are substantial.

Those changes won't happen here! The community loses its hospital due to the failure to hear the tsunami warnings.

What are you going to give us in return for our loyalty! A physician group holds its independence higher than its survival by refusing to work in a collaborative way with other physicians intent on changing operations.

We don't need any outsiders telling us what to do! The community mobilizes against the decision of the local hospital board by refusing to seriously consider the hospital's opportunity to join a network of health care facilities so that it can maintain its independence.

We've done it this way for years and it's worked, so why change now! Mental health professionals fail to respond to the calls for outpatient, not inpatient, services in caring for clients,

The thinking of customers is critical as a perspective on the components of the *operational triad* of infrastructure, strategy, and process as well as the *philosophical triad* of vision, mission, and values. The successful turnaround requires that the leader not only consider but also incorporate the thinking of the customer into the framework of analysis in preparing the turnaround plan. Questions to consider include:

■ Will the services continue if the organization fails?

■ What will be the impact on care and customers' perceptions of care if the turnaround is not successful?

■ How do I want the organization to change to meet customers' future needs?

Governance. The role of governance is especially crucial in a turnaround situation. It is totally insufficient to simply designate a turnaround leader and then proceed to get out of the way. Governance must be involved.

The responsibilities of governance in a turnaround include defining clear parameters on the degree of change that will be allowed in the turnaround, active involvement in core decisions involving restructuring and reengineering, embracing the vision and mission statements, supporting difficult changes publicly and politically, and taking risks with leadership and management leading the turnaround effort. Reactions to the turnaround by members of governance often make the difference between success and failure.

Those changes won't happen here! The board relies on past successes of the organization as the retaining wall for holding back the tides of a tsunami.

What are you going to give us in return for our loyalty! The board consists of members who have served for more than 15 years and who feel that discussions of change are an insult to their commitment and loyalty.

We don't need any outsiders telling us what to do! The board and its finance committee believe that the organization is unique and that past efforts to bring about change will not work now because they have been tried and have failed.

We've done it this way for years and it's worked, so why change now! The building committee develops a long-range plan for replacement of the acute care facility's plant.

Governance must ask serious questions and maintain active involvement, especially in the formative stages of the turnaround. Questions to consider include:

- What are our responsibilities in the turnaround?
- How did we contribute to the turnaround situation?
- What support can we offer leadership and management as the turnaround continues?
- What is our obligation to customers?

Leadership. Probably the single most important element of the successful turnaround is the leader! We can think of no other factor that will dictate the success or failure of a turnaround effort more than the person who is selected for the leadership role.

In Chapter V, a self–assessment was detailed. Turnarounds, *a priori*, require a certain baseline of attributes, skills, knowledge, and experiences. The six most critical skills of the effective turnaround leader tie directly to the six turnaround principles:

Simultaneity. Leaders who are incapable of dealing with multiple demands originating from different sources and with differing priorities will be thwarted in their efforts to lead a turnaround situation.

Rapidity. Because turnarounds demand accelerated decision making and change to recreate the organization, a unique leadership pace is required, especially in the formative stages. In our experience, the pace cannot be sustained over protracted periods except through extra-human effort.

Complexity. Complexity evolves from the requirement that the leader manage the old organization while defining a vision for the new entity, blending the two into a coherent framework for those who are assisting in creating the new order.

Uncertainty. Decisions in turnarounds never seem to be black or white. The grey zone dominates. The leader often is faced with pioneering new concepts for the organization that provide no guarantee of their effectiveness for the turnaround effort.

Management by Intuition. The ability to intuitively make demanding, simultaneous, rapid decisions in complex and uncertain situations is an imperative in the turnaround.

Leader Objectivity. Facing the turnaround with an objective, unbiased perspective remains a critical characteristic of the successful turnaround leader.

The leader must champion the turnaround! Without leadership, all other efforts within the organization will flounder. Examples of leadership perspectives that are unacceptable and their potential consequences include:

The changes won't happen here! After 20 years of leading the organization through growth and program development, the leader states emphatically that the community is immune to the changes in other markets because of its special situation.

What are you going to give me in return for my loyalty? If I can hang on just a little longer, I'll be able to retire out of this mess.

We don't need any outsiders telling us what to do! The IPA board doesn't need someone to give them special consulting advice on our structure because, as the CEO, I know what to do.

We've done it this way for years and it's worked, so why change now? The CEO proclaims to his or her board, "All of the changes being proposed will be more disruptive than maintaining a steady course."

The leader must ask any number of questions to validate his or her efforts in sustaining the turnaround effort. In addition to questions related to the organization, there are also personal questions that must be addressed if the leader is to be successful.

- How can I generate support for the turnaround effort?
- Will I survive?
- What are my responsibilities to governance? To customers? To management?
- Does everyone understand the severity of the situation?

Management. Turnaround leaders will be unsuccessful without the support, involvement, and commitment of key management staff. In many situations, management staff must be recruited from the outside rather than promoted from within because the transformational response required in a turnaround situation needs new creative energy. By recruiting external management for key positions, the leader is assured of support from individuals with high commitment and little historical investment in past practices of the organization. These attributes are necessary elements in providing support to the leader.

In addition to the turnaround leader, others are also crucial in fostering the turnaround effort. Cultivating leadership among staff is a difficult yet essential task if the turnaround is to be successful. Management reactions and associated risks include:

Those changes won't happen here! The senior management team fails to engage in asking difficult questions about the future of the organization, as well as about it's changing role.

What are you going to give us in return for our loyalty? The focus of the department is on the structure of the bonus payment rather than on the strategy for the turnaround effort.

We don't need any outsiders telling us what to do! Department heads are too busy to work with the organizational development consultant because of the press of other "more substantive" problems facing them.

We've done it this way for years and it's worked, so why change now? The chief financial officer believes that if the hospital refuses to engage in discussions with payers about their desire to implement a capitated product, the organization will be successful in limiting managed care growth in the market.

Managers who remain and those who come on board need to assess the turnaround situation and consider their roles in support of it. Critical questions that must be considered by the management team include:

- How can I support leadership in managing the turnaround process?
- What happens to me personally and professionally if the turnaround is successful? Unsuccessful?
- Who should I trust in guiding the turnaround effort?
- What are the limitations of the organization in meeting turnaround objectives?

Finally, in considering turnarounds, we have come to the conclusion that cautions for all critical stakeholders are important. Whether the turnaround is in business or health care, these cautions are critical to making a turnaround happen. Ignoring them can have devastating results! We urge you to consider them carefully within the context of the situation you intend to manage!

 CAUTION: *The Previous Leader Must Be Disempowered.*

Attempting a turnaround where the prior leader continues can, at a minimum, be difficult, if not impossible. The presence of the previous leader in a turnaround situation can be very destructive. Most frequently, the directions instituted by the previous leader are questioned and changed. If the previous leader remains in the organization and is resistant, he or she will undermine your efforts to make the needed changes

 CAUTION: *The Situation Often gets Worse Before It Gets Better, and the Organization May Not Have Hit Bottom Yet.*

Turnaround, by definition, means that an organization is in a major period of decline or is about to *hit bottom*. It is best to try and begin the turnaround before

hitting bottom, because, after that stage, it may be more difficult to mobilize the requisite resources for the turnaround effort. Also, it is important for the leader to understand that, if the organization has not hit bottom, he or she will be the leader when it does hit bottom! As a result, in the eyes of some, things get worse (apparently) before they get better. A good approach to build confidence in the capabilities of the leader is to articulate this phenomenon before it occurs.

 CAUTION: *Precipitate Decline or Collapse Can Be a Good Place to Be.*

Gradual, slow declines often blind those who are involved into a sense of complacency. Precipitate declines, however, result in a near panic state, where the organization realizes it must change or it will not survive. The state of decline can be very motivating to the governance and the staff of an organization. Take advantage of their willingness to cooperate.

 CAUTION: *Governance Must Be Totally Committed to a Change, Including Reconstitution of the Organization.*

For a turnaround to become reality, the support of governance or some other similar group is essential. Without their unswerving support, the leader attempting change will face mutiny, particularly as the organization hits bottom. Governance's role is to support the leader's vision and strategy of change.

 CAUTION: *People Will Not Be in the Same Place at the Same Time.*

Because of the nature of the turnaround situation, the people of the organization are on a spectrum of commitment to the changes happening to the organization. Some believe they are absolutely necessary; others question the changes but go along; still others perceive change as unnecessary. Most organizations have a spectrum of commitment; the difference with a turnaround is the breadth of the spectrum.

 CAUTION: *Expect Resistance.*

Change implies there will be resistance. Furthermore, the relationship is direct: the greater the change, the greater the resistance.

CAUTION: There Will Be Winners and Losers.

The inevitable characteristic of a turnaround is change. In any change, there are perceived winners and losers. It is not infrequent to have 100 percent turnover of top managers in a turnaround situation.

CAUTION: Thick Skin Is a Necessity, Because Thin Skin Is Easily Bruised and Lacerated.

Not all changes will be viewed as positive. People within the organization will have vested interests in maintaining the status quo. There will be difficult and painful moments in the organization's change that will directly affect the leader. It is critical to not personalize the situation and to stay above the near panic state that can occur in the formative stage of a turnaround. As noted above, there will always be winners and losers in a turnaround situation. A "this is business" mentality will help the turnaround leader survive.

CAUTION: Be Wary of People Bearing Gifts.

Frequently, those who are first in line and bearing gifts are the ones who need to go first. Be careful of the invitations for dinner, weekends at the cabin, and other "gifts." A turnaround may require that you terminate your host within weeks of the special event in your honor. At the same time, it's important to listen to all sources in the formative stage. It's tough, but, then again, it's a turnaround. This is not as cold-hearted as it sounds. It is simply a recognition of reality.

CAUTION: Turnarounds Do Not Occur without Sufficient Resources.

One of the major limitations in turnaround efforts is the lack of resources, both human and fiscal, dedicated to the turnaround. The need for such resources should never be underestimated. Furthermore, getting the best help at the worst time often entails an investment and remuneration above the norm, or at least with some rewards at the end of the tunnel. A pecuniary approach in the heat of battle engenders little support. At the same time, the watchwords for the leader must be appropriate investments.

CAUTION: *Keep Key Governance Leadership Informed on the Turnaround Effort.*

Too often, after the formative stage of the turnaround, the leader tends to neglect governance. Also, some turnaround situations require so much attention to putting out fires that the seemingly less important task of "reporting" can simply be put aside for other more pressing concerns. Neglect of governance at this stage, however, will come back to haunt the leader. Once again, it is important to stay above the fray and remember that, without support of governance, there is no turnaround!

 CAUTION: *People Want to Help—Listen Carefully and with Scrutiny.*

In a turnaround situation, you can rarely predict where the best ideas will germinate. Employees in the trenches often have a lot of ideas that will help the turnaround effort. Too frequently, they are the last to be asked. A good strategy is to listen to everyone. Serve as your own sieve for information. Rely upon the management team to help you assess the data and information, but also rely upon your managerial instincts.

 CAUTION: *It's Scary and Lonely*

One of the most difficult issues for the leader is that, during the formative stage of a turnaround, there are few people from whom you can seek counsel who are internal to the organization—especially if you're coming in from the outside. This is not paranoia; it's simply a state of reality. It is very frequently unclear in the formative stage what human resource changes are necessary to successfully complete the turnaround. Don't underestimate the need to develop and utilize support systems!

Chapter VII

The Question of
Infrastructure

Resources for Results

"Americans can always be relied upon to do the right thing, after they have exhausted all other possibilities."

Sir Winston Churchill

The Clean Up Begins

Infrastructure is the essential function in the turnaround model and the foundation of any turnaround effort. Without basic capacity, any turnaround effort is doomed to failure no matter how much determination, brilliance, or vision is instilled into the organization by the leader. In Chapter IV, we provided a series of questions to assist the leader in initiating a diagnostic assessment of the organization. The answers to several of these questions provide good insight into the prior infrastructure of the organization.

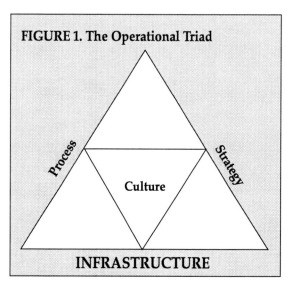

FIGURE 1. The Operational Triad

Process

Strategy

Culture

INFRASTRUCTURE

Six basic dimensions constitute the core infrastructure.

Space. The question of space available to an organization can be a crucial consideration in a turnaround. For example, in an environment where the demand for services is increasingly of an ambulatory nature, is it feasible to deliver health care in an institution designed with private beds under Hill-Burton specifications? Probably not. And yet many of us are trying to do just that! The space dilemma is a particularly acute problem for many smaller and rural facilities despite the availability of space in the form of unutilized beds. Available space is no space if it's not the right space.

Furthermore, it is increasingly recognized that the functionality of space dramatically affects operational costs, efficiency, and productivity—important variables in an increasingly capitated or fixed payment environment. The critical elements of space include:

■ Condition
■ Appearance
■ Functionality
■ Flexibility
■ Customer sensitivity
■ Geographic proximity
■ Convenience
■ Utility
■ Potential for modification

Equipment. Multiple issues exist around equipment in any health care institution. Equipment is particularly vexing for the leader, because it is too often used as a proxy for power and quality within the health care setting. Physicians like their toys!

The other major dilemma related to equipment is its ever-shortening span of usefulness before new and emerging technologies come to market. Each scanning device is seemingly outdated the moment it is placed into service because of new technological innovations. Critical equipment considerations include:

- Age
- Condition
- Functionality
- Utility
- Flexibility
- Upgradability

Information and Information Systems. Information is considered by many to be the most critical future issue in health care. Without information, determining the status of cost, quality, and effectiveness of the health care delivered by the organization is simply not feasible. Turnarounds by their very nature demand good information on the current status of the organization. Sustainable organizations that emerge from the turnaround situation are driven by information. Information is the core of the new health care system.

For example, in a managed care environment where an organization is attempting to transition from strictly managing access to effective care management at the point of service between the provider and the patient, information becomes the key variable for determining ultimate success. Managing access requires data on what was done. By whom. For what purpose. In what setting. With what results. Care management, on the other hand, requires information on process, outcomes, potential clinical choices, and most effective treatment methodologies. Furthermore, the information needs to be available to all providers in all settings at all times. If such an approach is not taken, the organization is almost forced to revert to an aggressive access management approach as a default in providing health care. Information systems considerations include:

- Flexibility
- Availability
- Responsiveness
- Accuracy
- Potential to grow
- Utilization
- Functionality
- User interface

Agreements and Contracts. The nature and type of agreements and contracts that exist within the organization can have a major impact on its ability to sustain a turnaround effort. These issues are particularly insidious in their effect on an organizational turnaround because they often extend far into the future. Also, agreements and contracts are frequently outside the control of the leader, especially in the formative stages of the turnaround.

Managed care contracts with physicians that include few incentives for resource management and utilization compliance can be major obstacles to any attempt to rebuild the infrastructure of an organization. Another example could include union contracts that block any attempts by leadership to launch reengineering or downsizing initiatives. Elements of agreements and contracts include:

- Length
- Buyout provisions
- Productivity stipulations
- Consistency with future organizational needs
- Limitations
- Negotiability

Human Resources. The ultimate turnaround asset is the human resources of an organization. Without people, an organization is simply a ship in dry dock with tsunamis on the horizon. True leaders recognize that mobilization of people is a far more compelling and effective resource for change than any vision statement or reorganization plan.

The difficulty with human resource considerations in a turnaround situation is separating the wheat from the chaff. Most organizations in need of a turnaround have outstanding individuals in the trenches who have been stifled in their ability to grow or contribute to change-oriented management decisions. Finding these individuals is a key first-step responsibility of the turnaround leader.

At the same time, the leader must identify employees who are not contributing to a successful turnaround effort. The lack of participation may be due to motivation, but it is more frequently due to lack of skills, abilities, and knowledge needed to sustain the new organizational state. Human resource considerations include:

- Number
- Type
- Capability
- Qualifications
- Experience
- Skills
- Training
- Capacity for change
- Competence
- Energy

Structure. How the organization is structured, both formally and informally, can result in significant repercussions for the turnaround. If an organization is structured properly, the functions needed to create and manage requisite changes can be accomplished in a timely, effective manner. This will facilitate the organization's growth and viability despite its vulnerability in a turnaround situation.

Medical schools are a prime example of institutions facing large turnaround imperatives. Most medical schools continue to be organized around the federation concept. Under such an approach, each department reigns as an independent entity. These individual fiefdoms result in high resource consumption, complex management, and needless duplication in an era of constraints requiring collaboration to maximize available resources. For example, too many departments in medical schools develop independent research initiatives, disconnected curricular programs, and independent communication efforts that will be difficult to sustain in the future. Elements of structure include:

- Line versus matrix
- Formal versus informal
- Hierarchical versus flat
- Rigid versus flexible
- Reporting relationships
- Functions
- Decision-making processes
- Empowerment

Summation

The final step on the question of infrastructure should be a definitive assessment of each component. It is crucial that these elements be considered together rather than in a singular fashion. Testament to the problems that can be created without systems thinking on infrastructure is evident throughout the health care system.

Consider the relation of space to information systems. Health care organizations bent on facing the new challenges of the coming health care environment have been known to spend millions on the design of ambulatory outpatient facilities that did not include computerized physician workstations.

Another example is the interface between client-centered care (i.e., structure) and the traditional hospital (i.e., space). Promoting a client-centered philosophy and approach to the delivery of services can be exceedingly difficult with long corridors, distant storage sites, inconvenient records accessibility, and other obstacles to care.

The question of infrastructure is crucial in the turnaround situation. As the foundation of the turnaround model, it deserves careful attention and focus by the leader.

CHAPTER VIII

A Question
of Finances

It's Not the Money, It's the Money

*"Certainly there are lots of things in life that money won't buy,
but it is very funny—Have you ever tried to buy them without money?"*

*Ogden Nash
"The Terrible People"—Happy Days, 1933*

Investing in the Future
by Raymond H. Barton III

Whether we like it or not, health care is a business. In a capitalistic society, currency and capital are not only the means to conduct commerce, but also how we "keep score." In the preceding chapter, we discussed the major elements related to infrastructure. A subset of infrastructure that is vital to any turnaround effort is the question of finances.

Thomas Jefferson was one of the few founding fathers who seemed to understand this principle fully. As one of the authors of the Declaration of Independence and of the U.S. Constitution, Jefferson was a "creator" of the balance of power among the three branches of government. However, Jefferson is said to have observed, after the constitution was approved, that if one really wanted to know where power in America would be based, one should "follow the power of the purse."

When this principle is applied to *The Turnaround Imperative*, the following concept has served as a helpful guide in many difficult discussions and political situations: "Remember, it doesn't matter what they're talking about. They're talking about money." This may be the single most important message to keep in mind during a turnaround. On the surface, this message may seem to suggest that mission, vision, values, the needs of the stakeholders, and humanitarian issues are less important than money. Quite the contrary. Remembering that "they're talking about money" helps to:

■ Avoid confusion in communication.

■ Meet the spoken and unspoken requirements of your partners.

■ Recognize that, in a capital-based society, you must address the issue of resources.

■ Acknowledge that, in order to meet the organization's mission and vision, resources and financial success are required.

Addressing Finances: Cookbook versus Principles

The most typical question asked by turnaround leaders is: What steps do I follow in successfully leading a financial turnaround? In other words, they want a cookbook, allowing them to simply follow the printed steps until they have successfully baked a cake (achieved financial success). Unfortunately, there is no such cookbook. If there were, turnaround leadership would not be needed.

In Chapter II, the *Principle of Management by Intuition* was introduced as one of the most vital personal strengths in successful turnaround leadership. There is no question that the top achievers have mastered this management trait and that it is a skill that is extremely difficult to teach. Contrary to popular belief, nowhere is

Raymond H. Barton III serves as President/CEO of St. Joseph's Health Care System, Albuquerque, New Mexico. Ray has extensive finance experience in turnaround situations.

the use of intuition more valuable than in the area of finances. However, there are several management initiatives and lessons that can be very useful in achieving success in the financial turnaround. They can be divided into five categories:

■ Strategy Meets Finance
■ Assets
■ Liabilities
■ Structure
■ Surfing Successes

Strategy Meets Finance

Doing the right thing. As mentioned in Chapters VI and IX, developing new strategic directions that must be pursued in the turnaround is critical. The effort will be ineffective, however, unless adequate financial resources are identified and committed by the organization to the turnaround effort. Peter Drucker put it very well in his statement: "Nothing is less productive than to make more efficient that which should not be done at all."

Therefore, the first rule of financial management is to ensure that the right strategic direction is being financed. Otherwise, precious resources and time are expended on something that will have to be undone and redone.

Quality is a financial endeavor. In a similar way, lack of quality costs. The cost of undoing and/or redoing something is typically much higher than simply doubling the cost of doing it right the first time. This is particularly true in health care, where poor quality not only has a negative effect in the business community, but can also have severe financial repercussions in the medical liability arena.

Assets

Cash is king—short-term considerations. When a serious turnaround situation is identified, the organization is typically in a well-established "death spiral." One reason for this situation is that management has a great deal of flexibility in reporting the results of operations on the income statement (statement of revenues and expenses). This flexibility comes from the ability to manipulate reserves on the balance sheet from a conservative position (high reserves) to a liberal position (low reserves).

In a similar way, insufficient cash flows and/or funding of depreciation can also be masked in two ways. First, these are balance sheet reporting functions and there is often a poor understanding of the balance sheet, even in financial circles. Second, short-term borrowing and/or restructuring of debt can be used to demonstrate average to high cash balances, even though the organization's operations are not generating the cash necessary to fund its capital needs.

As a result of these two masking devices, companies are usually well along the disaster pathway before the seriousness of the situation becomes obvious. Because management has a career stake in this process, it is not unusual for the board of directors to finally step in and initiate the turnaround. By this time, cash and the borrowing flexibility of the organization are typically measured on a day-to-day basis. Therefore, finding short-term capital is clearly a financial imperative.

So, where do you go for short-term capital? Dillinger, the outlaw, had the answer for us. When asked why he robbed banks, he replied, "Because that's where the money is." The same logic applies in seeking capital for a turnaround situation. For short-term capital, we need to go where the money is. In doing so, it is important to realize that we may not be seeking a true source of long-term capital but rather the use of capital to help the organization through its short-term capital crisis.

In health care, federal and state governments are clearly "where the money is." Government programs continue to be the dominant financing mechanisms for health care services in this country. In addition, the government has well-defined rules that govern capital floats (i.e., who owes money to whom). Therefore, one of the very first activities that should be undertaken in an organization that has been poorly operated is to completely review any open financial filings with government programs. In many turnaround situations, this has resulted in an amended filing and a reversal of the capital float.

Cash is king—long-term considerations. Unlike the general business world, health care organizations have typically lived by their financial statements. This means that management is usually judged by the results reported on the income statement (i.e., yearly profits). The problem is that the profits reported on the income statement may or may not translate into cash and cash equivalents, which are reported on the balance sheet. In contrast, the management of publicly traded companies is typically judged by two criteria:

- Cash earnings per share
- Value per share (a function of earnings per share and the balance sheet strength of the company)

The key concept is that health care organizations have ignored the balance sheet for too long. Once short-term stability is achieved, the turnaround leader must initiate the process of educating governance and the broader management team on the value of strengthening the organization's balance sheet, for long-term organizational stability. Balance sheet improvements and ratio analyses should be occasion for celebration and commendation, just as positive profit results are...perhaps even more so.

Liabilities

Entitlements. As the federal government has learned in trying to balance the budget, if you don't control entitlements, all other financial efforts may be in vain. Entitlements are built-in commitments and associated costs that the organization has to people and/or other organizations to which the latter are entitled. These may or may not be tied to the financial performance of the organization. Examples of entitlements in health care organizations are retirement contributions and policies, programs to increase base salary levels and/or benefit levels based on employee tenure, termination benefits, and/or policies protecting employment (such as in downsizing or layoffs).

Entitlements are present in any organization and are often both a surprise to management and a serious financial setback when an effort to downsize the organization begins. Employment and benefit policies that were established in the more moderate days of health care have usually not been rewritten in years or even decades. Even in preparation for accreditation reviews, personnel and management policies are often simply retyped and reapproved as is.

Policies/entitlements that deserve special attention at the very beginning of a turnaround are found in the following areas:

- Employment-at-will issues.
- Termination rights and benefits, particularly notice periods, appeal rights, and payout requirements based on tenure.
- Disciplinary policies and employee rights (this is particularly important in light of the need to set new standards of performance).
- Compensation and evaluation policies.
- Merit versus tenure rewards.
- Market versus internally driven compensation structure.
- Officers and directors liability coverage and indemnity policies.

Contracts and agreements. An old adage states: "What you don't know can't hurt you." In the case of prior contracts and agreements that the organization has entered into, however, the opposite of this statement is true. Liabilities from previous contracts/agreements tend to surface during these times of change, when you can least afford it. As a result, it is very wise to invest time in a review of all significant contracts and agreements.

There are basically two types of contracts/agreements: formal and informal. Formal contracts will typically not be found in one place. Health care organizations have traditionally divided responsibility for contracts by service, with financial, medical, materials management, food service, physical plant, volunteers, foundation, and managed care contracts often being based in different locations. A good rule of thumb is that, in a turnaround situation, you will almost always find contracts that are a surprise to someone in senior management.

Informal agreements are obviously more difficult to identify and review. They are identified only through conversations with individuals who are in key management/physician relationship positions. There will almost always be several informal agreements, particularly commitments to physicians, that will be very painful to honor. There will be pressure within the management team and sometimes even within governance not to honor these types of commitments. It is imperative to honor these agreements, however, once it is verified that they are valid. The new leadership team's credibility in financial and operational commitments is often determined by how past commitments of the organization are honored or discarded. If any agreement is so onerous as to jeopardize the future of the organization, the parties should be notified of that fact, all information should be shared with them, and a request should be made to renegotiate the agreement.

One last principle involving the review of liabilities relates to "physician giveaways," usually by hospital-based organizations. In conducting a review of both entitlements and contracts/agreements, unreasonable physician giveaways will often surface. These are financial or beneficial commitments made by health care organizations to select physicians that are clearly unfair, unreasonable, unethical, and/or illegal under the heat of current review. Nearly all hospitals have made such deals in the past, and many are still paying for them.

If such agreements are uncovered, it is usually very wise to address them directly with the physician or physicians involved and very early in the turnaround. The primary reason for such urgency is that, in the early days of a significant financial turnaround, there is much greater support for the big things that need to be done to save the organization. This is particularly true in regard to governance, where support is often needed in dealing with sensitive physician issues.

Structure

The budget: To redo or not to redo? The question of whether to restate the organization's operating budget is always a difficult one. The answer may be a function of how much of the fiscal year remains when the turnaround effort is initiated.

There is nothing wrong with resetting the budget on the basis of a new set of operating expectations and strategic directions. However, there are two principles to remember in making this decision:

■ The budget process is difficult and time-consuming for all of management. However, for the staff of the financial areas, it is nearly an all-consuming process during the active stages. The decision must therefore be made as to the cost-benefit ratio of having management and finance staffs focusing on a paper document versus focusing on reinventing management and operations.

■ More and more often, high achievers in management express concern regarding reliance on the budgeting process as a primary means of managing an organization. For example, Jack Welch, CEO of General Electric, believes that budgets are like "handcuffs, which actually limit managers' performance and hold down higher profits." In the brave new world of health care, leaders should be open to new ways of measuring and managing organizational success.

Budget set-asides. In Chapter IV, the ideas involved in investing in research and development (R&D), as well as in identification of future core businesses, were presented. In the early days of a major turnaround, identifying and funding resources for future core businesses (i.e., the vision) is one of the most difficult tasks imaginable. Even if the organization's new turnaround enjoys exceptional visionary and communication skills, creating budget set-asides for such invisible objectives seems a little crazy, even to yourself. And if it seems a little crazy to you, imagine how it sounds to middle managers or physician partners who are being asked to make serious financial and personal sacrifices.

Regardless, one of the most visible indicators of a true turnaround leader is commitment to budget set-asides for future development. This is particularly true in the early days of a turnaround. In the beginning of a financial turnaround, much of the needed capital will be found in cost-cutting. However, earlier than is typically comfortable, the focus will turn to how the new leadership is generating fresh marketplace initiatives and revenues (or the lack thereof). If an investment in future initiatives has been made from day one, success in R&D is greatly enhanced.

Organizational controls and attention to detail. In the formative stages of a turnaround, the leader serves multiple roles. In addition to being CEO, the person is chief financial officer (CFO) and chief information officer (CIO). As a result, control and approval thresholds should be moved up in the organization. Senior management, particularly the CEO, should be involved in virtually everything involving control decisions. Being involved in this level of approval detail creates three benefits (all of which are positive if they are not left in place for too long):

- By its very nature, this process creates bureaucracy, which tends to slow down cash outflows by slowing the approval process.
- Because supervisors and management are aware that submissions will receive closer review, the number of nonessential requests is diminished.
- Senior management very quickly learns a great deal about how the organization works.

Financial Structure

Improperly structuring financial departments is a common mistake in turnaround situations. Very often, the CFO is turned into a financial monster. The CEO designates the CFO as the "hatchetman," responsible to identify and eliminate employees/functions that can be cut from the organization. By negatively stereotyping the financial staff, a key staff resource is cut off from the rest of the organization's employees. This isolation and/or fear can extend to the medical staff as well. The most damaging part of this early reputation is that it is nearly impossible to reverse later, when you need the financial staff to work in concert with everyone else.

In the most difficult days of a turnaround, if the new CEO and senior management are willing to also fulfill the hard-line CFO functions, it frees the CFO and other financial staff members to become a very valuable resource to all of management. The CFO becomes accessible to management as a supportive staff resource, helping to realign budgets, projects, requests, priorities, and strategic planning initiatives, rather than being feared and avoided at all costs.

Setting new performance standards. Perhaps the most important leadership function, to be initiated on day one, is establishment of new and higher financial standards for the entire organization. Not only must this occur on day one, but also on every day thereafter until the turnaround is complete! It should always be noted that these new standards are in effect for everyone, including the CEO. As was noted earlier, expectations are a very powerful tool in achieving greater financial and operational results. It seems to be a truism that people tend to meet the expectations that are set for them.

In addition to the reward of having the entire organization begin to march to a faster beat, there is a very practical reason for formally communicating the setting of new standards. This relates back to the section of this chapter dealing with liabilities. Whenever major employment policies are replaced by new ones, significant financial and legal liabilities are a possibility. Therefore, by communicating that previous expectations and standards of the organization are being raised and that each employee (including senior management) will be evaluated and governed by those new, higher standards from this day forward, two fundamental objectives are met:

■ Legal documentation is created, establishing the new standards and why they are necessary and reasonable. Unfortunately, in our society, such liability-reducing actions are necessary to protect the organization.

■ Employees deserve clear and specific communication regarding organizational expectations, individual performance, employment policies, and measurement standards. This approach both is fair to employees and demonstrates open communication to the entire team.

Surfing Successes

The turnaround begins through the creation and selling of a new organizational vision. President Ronald Reagan, nicknamed "The Great Communicator," is a prime example of a leader who was able to articulate a new vision for America. Creating excitement and buy-in for a new vision will typically generate enough positive movement to start the organizational turnaround.

However, there comes a time (which is different in every turnaround) when rhetoric must turn to actual, measurable results. In most settings, a universally accepted measurement of results is financial success. Therefore, it is a wise leadership team that maps out one or two demonstration projects that can be used to demonstrate early financial success for the redirected organization. Ironically, these surfing successes do not need to be very large in scale. However, they do need to be in areas that are considered strategic to the new organizational vision. It also helps if they are in areas involving health care services, rather than support or business services.

Properly planned and managed, these surfing successes will be remembered long after one would have thought their importance would be diminished. This is particularly true in the medical community. Remember: Reputations are won early and can last a lifetime.

CHAPTER IX

Steps in the Management
of Strategy and Process

The How of Turnarounds

*"There are many institutions in history that have simply
winked out of existence because there was no need for them anymore.
Where's the nearest watermill?"*

James Burke

The Framework for Rebuilding

In addition to infrastructure, the operational triad includes attention to strategy and process. In Chapter VI, strategy was defined as containing two elements. The first is internally focused and involves activities applied by the leader to the management of the turnaround. The second element is externally focused and involves development of new strategic directions concerning the organization's future. Both elements are deemed critical to a successful turnaround effort. The core elements of process were also highlighted. Without adequate considera-

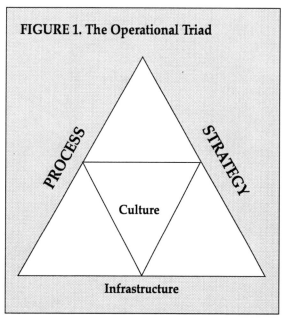

FIGURE 1. The Operational Triad

tion of group dynamics, overt and covert behaviors, interpersonal relationships organizational norms, and other process issues, the turnaround effort will be jeopardized.

So, let's get started! There are a number of crucial actions that the turnaround leader must undertake to be successful. We recommend that you approach the strategies and processes outlined in this chapter in a relatively linear way, while continuing to recognize the six turnaround principles of simultaneity, rapidity, complexity, uncertainty, management by intuition, and leader objectivity.

 ACTION: *Understand the human side of change and your role as a change agent.*

The nature of a turnaround is to be objective, decisive, rapid, and strategic, yet to ignore the human side of change could eventually undermine your long-term success.

First, to be sensitive to the human side of change, it must be understood. People's reactions to the magnitude of change that will be required by the turnaround may spell the end of life as they knew it, and they will treat this as a major loss. Just as with a loved one who dies, they will go through the cycle of loss:

- **Denial and disbelief:** *It must be a mistake!*
- **Anger and attack:** *I can't believe how they're destroying this place!*
- **Bargains and deals:** *If we slow down, wouldn't things go better?*
- **Depression and sadness:** *Everything I've worked on is in jeopardy!*
- **Acceptance and resolution:** *Well, maybe he's right after all.*

The cycle of loss will play out in the early days of the turnarounds. It is important that they are recognized as normal. Sometimes it is sufficient just to recognize how people are feeling and to not overreact.

At the same time, the leader must be aware that, if people are stuck somewhere in the cycle, it may be necessary to intervene in a more direct way to move them forward. Some people will never let go of the past or move beyond denial and anger. Helping them leave the organization is probably necessary. It also is a clear signal for those remaining about their need for commitment and acceptance.

 Action: Identify the critical players and schedule interviews with them.

One of the most important initial tasks for the turnaround leader is to identify the internal and external people critical to managing the turnaround. All key stakeholders must be interviewed by the turnaround leader, including board members, external stakeholders, managerial staff, and executive leadership. Also, never underestimate the power of the secretary or executive assistant in providing insight into the situation. He or she may have more insight into the problems you are facing than executives, who will no doubt be anticipating actions by the leader, that may jeopardize their situation. Seeking candor is the name of the game!

Make a list of everyone you can identify for the initial series of interviews. After the first series of interviews, the major stakeholders of the organization who are critical to the turnaround will have been identified.

There are basically five questions to ask each person during the interviews:

- What do you believe will turn the organization around? Why?
- What are the barriers to accomplishing the turnaround?
- How can you help me with the turnaround?
- What are the three things I can do for you over the next three months as we work together to make the turnaround happen?
- What three people should I contact to assess the organizational situation?

Keep the interview simple and listen carefully! It is equally important to interview known creators, supporters, skeptics, and saboteurs (see discussion later in this chapter). Identifying those who do not believe in the need for a turnaround can be difficult, but it is important. These interviews will be one of the most important activities accomplished during the formative stages of the turnaround.

ACTION: *Involve the critical players in completing a thorough organizational assessment.*

Keep in mind the need to involve selected critical players in defining the organization's problem statement, assessment, and subsequent turnaround strategies. Involvement and investment by the critical players will increase their commitment to the turnaround effort. Chapter IV provides a framework and key questions for the organizational assessment.

As an example, the turnaround of a small rural hospital can be particularly tricky. In small towns, everyone knows everyone and everyone is involved with everyone. At the same time, everyone knows that everyone's involvement will not necessarily result in an effective turnaround. Who should attend an initial strategy retreat becomes an especially critical decision that will directly affect the success of the turnaround effort.

Each situation is different. In some cases, all members of the medical staff should be asked to attend. In others, involvement of physicians would spell disaster, especially if the invited individuals were key parts of the organization's decline.

Keep in mind that previously unrecognized leaders will often percolate to the top in a turnaround situation. Never underestimate the power of their support in the conduct of meetings and retreats where discussions on the organizational turnaround will evolve into commitment and involvement.

Also, in almost every turnaround situation, the assessment process will identify stakeholders who can be considered to be critical players but who in reality are opposed to change efforts and hold substantial differences with the turnaround strategy. In fact, by engaging them in the turnaround, they will actually "dig in their heels" and become increasingly opposed to the need for change. It is imperative to deal directly with these individuals early in the process.

ACTION: *Consider using external resources in assisting with the organizational assessment and in helping refine strategies and processes needed for the*

It is highly probable that external help will be needed in the formative stages of the turnaround. Don't hesitate to spend well-focused, and often scarce, financial resources for good consultative assistance. Areas that frequently require external technical assistance include infrastructure and facilities assessment, finance and capital requirements, third-party reimbursement methodologies, management and information systems, assessment of staff competencies, managed care approaches, and organizational development.

One of the most underutilized external consultants in the turnaround situation is in the area of organizational development. Frequently, organizational development consultants are viewed as soft on detail in an environment demanding definitive expertise. However, outside consultative expertise in organizational development is frequently at the heart of crafting a new vision and in helping to manage the key changes needed for success.

Identifying the organizational development consultant early in the overall process is a wise strategy. The consultant can serve in a behind-the-scenes or "shadow consultant" role. Later on, after the initial strategy and process are better defined, the organizational consultant can publicly assist the leader with key meetings and activities that directly facilitate involvement of staff, board members, and other external stakeholders.

 ACTION: *Prepare* The Memo.

Once the organizational assessment is completed and the magnitude of the changes required for the organization is well understood, we suggest that the turnaround leader prepare an initial memo or document—for him- or herself and for the board. *The Memo* is a critical first step in clarifying vision and direction, articulating needed changes, and generating support. *The Memo* should include certain key elements:

- **Assessment:** An assessment should be made of the reasons the organization is facing a turnaround situation. As noted previously, a brief overview of the business operations, financial status, leadership issues, human resource capabilities, and existing culture are key elements of this section.

- **Vision:** The leader's vision in the early stages of the turnaround is vital, although eventual buy-in by governance and other stakeholders is crucial. Where and why the leader wants to take the organization are critical elements that will guide future action. Initial reactions to the leader's vision should be carefully considered, as they are indications of people's readiness for and acceptance of needed changes.

- **Implementation Steps:** The first steps made in the turnaround process are often the most critical. Missteps or miscues will either elicit support or will build barriers to the turnaround among staff and management of the organization. A clear outline of what to do when, and how is an invaluable aid as the leader proceeds through the turnaround. At first, plan implementation steps in time frames no longer than 3-6 months duration.

- **Resource Needs:** No turnaround can be completed without sufficient resources. Key considerations are financial, human, and information resources. These need to be made very explicit in *The Memo* if the leader is to have a chance of acquiring needed resources.

In particular, *The Memo* can be used with governance and other key stakeholders concerning the state of the organization. *The Memo* is only your best estimate of what is needed, but it is critical to begin to build a commitment from governance and a shared game plan for immediate action.

 ACTION: *Schedule a series of retreats to facilitate a consensus on the vision, mission, values, strategy, and initial processes to be utilized during the formative stages of the turnaround.*

The complexity of the turnaround effort and the concurrent need for personal reeducation of staff and board members will necessitate extensive and focused discussion. Based on our experience, such work cannot be done at the office where myriad demands divert the focus of senior management. Rather, it requires a retreat atmosphere.

Retreats, while costly in terms of time, can actually be a much more time-efficient approach to creating consensus on direction for the organization. In many organizations, just getting people away from the office for a day signals a new way of working. The retreat, if directed by a skilled facilitator, can open up creative thinking on the part of the turnaround's most important asset—the people of the organization. We recommend that the leader not serve as the facilitator—even if he or she has substantial training. Active involvement and investment of the leader in the turnaround decisions is too crucial, and the leader cannot be a neutral, unbiased facilitator in group discussions. Serving as the facilitator requires neutrality—a trait for others, not the leader of the turnaround effort!

The number of retreats and the time frame required for a given turnaround situation will vary substantially. Insist on participation! Don't listen to those in the organization who insist that they don't have time for retreats. The effective retreat provides the setting for creating a new vision and strategy for the organization's survival—some of the most important work in which employees can be involved.

The first series of retreats should focus on the results of the organizational assessment and should begin to work on creating a consensus around the vision, mission, and values for the organization (see Chapter X). While a leader can initially define the vision, he or she must get everyone involved in *refining the vision*. While the mission may be obvious, unless it is stated there is no clear consensus. Values for one may not be the values for others. Consensus is absolutely essential.

Once there is consensus on the assessment and the vision for the organization is clear, the mission of the organization can be discussed and focused. It is not sufficient to just disseminate these documents to staff and assume that people will embrace them.

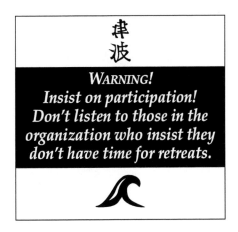

Achieving consensus and buy-in can only be accomplished by developing appropriate forums where people can understand, question, and even disagree with what is presented. These forums, whether they are one-hour meetings, brown-bag lunches, or half-day retreats, represent another mechanism for the turnaround leadership to be visible and to help everyone in the organization let go of the past and prepare for the future.

Often symbols can be crucial. One of the authors passed out coal ("I'm just an old lump of coal...") to every new employee and created the diamond (...but I'm gonna be a diamond someday") award for organizational accomplishments related to the vision and contributions to the turnaround effort. Similar analogies are often more useful than words in generating support and enthusiasm among the troops.

 ACTION: *Create an ongoing, formal process of team development for key players in the organization.*

The magnitude of the leadership requirements in managing a turnaround situation demands an investment in developing a team. Without the availability of a high-performing team, the demands of simultaneity, rapidity, complexity, uncertainty, management by intuition, and leader objectivity will overpower even the most seasoned leader. In particular, it is important to understand that teams have different functions for different purposes in different situations. There are many types of teams needed in the turnaround situation:

- **Leadership teams:** Set organizational policy, clarify vision and set mission, finalize turnaround assessment.
- **Cross-functional or interdisciplinary teams:** Cross-fertilize and integrate turnaround strategies across departments.
- **Management teams:** Coordinate and supervise, manage resources, set objectives.

- **Operational teams:** Solve problems, design processes for specific work units, work on continuous quality improvement.
- **Self-directed work teams:** Have responsibility and autonomy for day-to-day problem solving, develop policy implementation strategies.

Team development can be a time-consuming and difficult task. Developing a team for the sake of team development serves little purpose in a turnaround situation. Rather, it is important to develop teams that function around critical tasks within specified timelines. It is also important to delineate between team and individual accountability

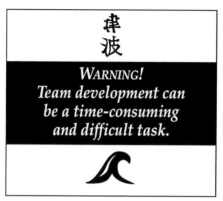

WARNING!
Team development can be a time-consuming and difficult task.

At the same time, it is important to recognize that well-functioning teams must possess requisite skills and resources. All too frequently, managers will assume that teams can function simply by being convened. Without training, without facilitation, without defining roles and goals, most teams will have difficulty functioning in any system, especially a turnaround.

One of the most effective approaches to team development is to combine the task of the team with needed training and support in an on-the-job training format. An external team development consultant or internal human resources or organizational development staff can be very helpful with this process. In such an approach, the consultant helps the team develop effective management skills and provides it with feedback, while simultaneously having the group work on the urgent tasks needed for the turnaround situation.

 ACTION: *Restructure the organization so that the newly minted mission, vision, values, and strategy can become a reality.*

Early in the turnaround effort, it is essential to examine the organization's structure and its effectiveness at accomplishing the turnaround. You can bet that the old organizational structure must be changed. It is based on a failing organization and, no doubt, is held together by individuals who are too frequently confined to the security of what they know best, rather than invested in the creation of what is best for the organization.

An important first step in restructuring the organization is to define the critical functions that must be managed and the skill set of the individuals managing those functions. If human resource issues are present in the organization, they will become evident during the organizational assessment.

The entire restructuring process can be very scary for the staff. A natural part of any restructuring is the inclusion or exclusion of people in the new structure. In fact, individuals who have been with the organization for a long time may need to be cut. Turnarounds are not for the faint of heart. The turnaround must, of necessity, at times reflect a public ruthlessness. The turnaround leader often experiences substantial personnel struggles that are extremely hard and difficult to manage. Not all staff will be severely affected, but all will need to at least think through how they will do their job differently based on *The Turnaround Imperative.*

 ACTION: *Implement internal change methodologies related to quality, reengineering, and structure.*

To assist the turnaround, a number of emerging internal change methodologies have begun to be utilized by health care organizations, including continuous quality improvement, total quality management, and reengineering. They can be particularly valuable, in that the approaches and tools used in these techniques help shift the organization toward a problem-solving approach to change. Furthermore, restructuring of internal processes is often an essential component of the larger turnaround effort.

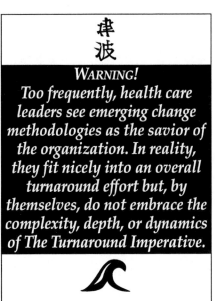

WARNING!
Too frequently, health care leaders see emerging change methodologies as the savior of the organization. In reality, they fit nicely into an overall turnaround effort but, by themselves, do not embrace the complexity, depth, or dynamics of The Turnaround Imperative.

ACTION: *Plot the possible behavioral responses to the turnaround and develop approaches to deal with them.*

Early on in the turnaround, both internal and external stakeholders will begin to exhibit behavior that either helps or hinders the turnaround. The turnaround leader must track these individuals from the beginning and develop specific approaches for managing the behaviors.

Behaviors will be manifested at multiple levels in the turnaround. It may relate to the process of a turnaround, the vision, the strategy, or a host of other dimensions that may affect individuals tied to the organization.

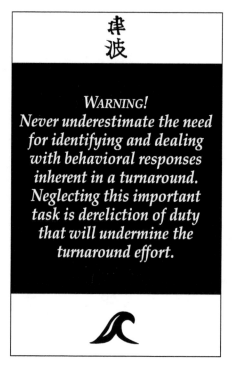

WARNING!
Never underestimate the need for identifying and dealing with behavioral responses inherent in a turnaround. Neglecting this important task is dereliction of duty that will undermine the turnaround effort.

The job of the turnaround leader is to explicitly identify the attributes of the people in the organization and to determine their degree of involvement and commitment to the turnaround. People tend to fall into four categories regarding their commitment and involvement: creators, supporters, skeptics, and saboteurs (see figure on page 83). Based on the results of the analysis, a specific approach for dealing with each person must be identified. By defining the degree of sabotage, skepticism, support, and creative energy for the turnaround effort, the leader will be able to allocate the limited time and resources of the organization. For each type of person, a three-pronged approach is:

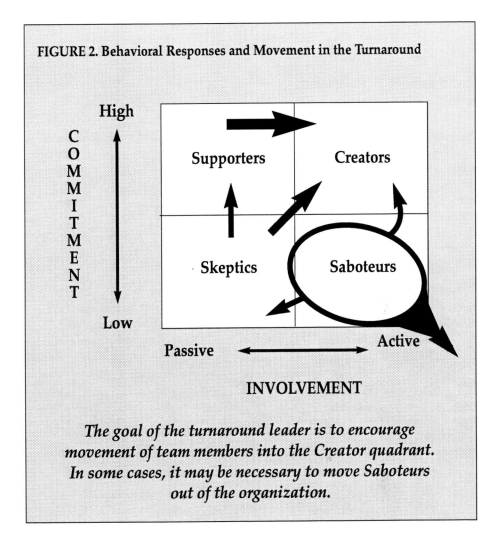

FIGURE 2. Behavioral Responses and Movement in the Turnaround

The goal of the turnaround leader is to encourage movement of team members into the Creator quadrant. In some cases, it may be necessary to move Saboteurs out of the organization.

- Share the vision, mission, strategy, structure, time schedule, and anticipated results of the turnaround.
- Determine the commitment level to and degree of involvement in the turnaround.
- Create a strategy to move everyone in a direction of creative involvement and high commitment to the turnaround.

Creators (Active Involvement/High Commitment): Creators are individuals in the organization who share the sense of vision, strategy, and timing required for the successful turnaround. These people demonstrate their support through active involvement in all facets of the turnaround. To sustain their support, the turnaround leader must:

- Treat them as confidential colleagues by sharing details on the turnaround process.
- Problem solve with them and use them as sounding boards in periods of uncertainty and doubt.
- Let them serve as surrogates in carrying the message forward, especially in areas where they exhibit or hold more credibility.
- Listen to their critiques and encourage feedback from them concerning your effectiveness as a leader.

Supporters (Passive Involvement/High Commitment): These people seem to be aligned with the stated vision and strategy and yet often are perceived as holding back their involvement in the turnaround. To elicit their support, the turnaround leader must:

- Acknowledge their support in public forums.
- Engage them in discussions about the importance of their roles in the future of the organization.
- Uncover their apprehensions and concerns about the implementation strategies of the turnaround.
- Determine what needs to be done organizationally to enlist them as creators.
- Give them important tasks to complete that will acknowledge their commitment to the turnaround process.

Skeptics (Passive Involvement/Low Commitment): These individuals hold strong, divergent opinions about the need for the turnaround. They are often articulate adversaries who need more information before coming aboard the turnaround effort. To enhance their commitment and involvement, the turnaround leader must:

- Understand the rationale for their skepticism, because it may be based on some historical reality.
- Recognize that their perspective can provide insight into the actions of those who may be taking more active, saboteur roles in the organization.
- Increase their degree of involvement and commitment to the turnaround effort through external education, inclusion in key meetings, and offering responsibility under a *quid pro quo* arrangement.

Saboteurs (Active Involvement/Low Commitment): These are the ultimate turnaround busters! It is often impossible to negotiate any degree of support for the turnaround effort. Furthermore, they frequently cannot be trusted even when confronted directly about issues, concerns, or plans. They frequently become actively involved in *opposition* to the turnaround effort. These people are often the most difficult and time-consuming to manage. Ultimately, they can endanger the success of the turnaround. To survive the saboteur, the turnaround leader must:

- Refuse to engage them in fundamental philosophical debates that are contrary to the reasons for the turnaround.

- Listen carefully and try to understand their views while concurrently determining their motives for undermining the turnaround effort.
- Create opportunities for the saboteurs to expose their views in front of others in the organization so that they have the opportunity to highlight their ideas as contrary to *The Turnaround Imperative*.
- Expect nothing positive from them in the early stages of the turnaround.
- Offer them opportunities that move them into another category, or be prepared to facilitate their exit from the organization quickly, if necessary!

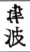 **ACTION:** *Implement formal and informal, internal and external, continuous scanning of the environment.*

Another important element of the ongoing process of a turnaround is the need for continuous scanning. The constant need to dangle your antennae in the winds of change cannot be stated strongly enough! Examples of activities important in this process include:

- Informal activities and events that facilitate communication among the members of the team are often an important strategy for obtaining information on the turnaround process (e.g., picnics, stop-bys, an open-door policy for specific hours of the week).
- Informal newsletters that include communication directly from the office of the CEO to the organization and that transmit real information on changes occurring in the organization can be invaluable.
- Formal, externally focused communication is also important (e.g., newsletter) in transmitting the directions and flavor of the "new" organization.
- Develop an external network of colleagues who are in similar situations or have turnaround experience so you can get some feedback on your ideas and progress.

In the early stages, the reliability of information is always suspect. There are several tips that will guide you in assessing the validity of information coming to you. First, do not reject any information for the first three months, regardless of the source. Second, those who knock on the door first may be least reliable as information sources. Third, rumors often run rampant during the first few months, so listen to them but do not react to them. Remembering these tips will help you sustain a scanning process that provides reliable, valid information on the status of the turnaround.

 ACTION: *Develop a budget that is consistent with the new direction of the organization.*

Aligned mission, vision, strategy, and structure are meaningless without support from the budget. The budget reflects the organizational allocation of resources and the emphasis of the turnaround effort. As discussed in Chapter VIII, the turnaround leader must eventually develop a totally new budget that reflects the new organization's needs. The failure to tie the budget to the new strategy and vision will not only slow down the turnaround effort but may even kill momentum in the formative stage.

Reallocation of funds away from old programs and activities to new ideas and ways of thinking is a powerful force for precipitating change. Furthermore, making the changes public garners the involvement and commitment of supporters and creators in the turnaround effort.

 ACTION: *Understand the complexity of change in health care and your role as a change agent.*

Critical to the success of the leader in a turnaround situation is an understanding of his or her role as a change agent. Many books have been written on this subject, but much less has been written on the change process as it relates to health care. Keep these points in mind as the turnaround evolves.

- *The focus of health professional education is on specialized functions that require independent, rather than interdependent, relationships.* Turnaround situations, *a priori*, require a breakdown of traditional barriers and the independent, singular, disciplinary thinking that ultimately thwart the process. We believe that turnarounds are simply not possible without a team approach!

- *As a rule, physicians are very smart, and yet they possess little education about business or the change processes inherent in turnaround situations.* Once again, the education of professionals interferes with their ability to become effective change agents. As a result, they frequently end up as either skeptics or saboteurs. Yet, if they can be shown that the changes will benefit them, rapid retooling can be the result.

- *The experience of most physicians in organized settings has been restricted to medical staffs, which function as constituency-based entities.* Constituency-based entities are often paralyzed by a process that requires consideration of every opinion and perspective. It is akin to the problems that would exist in the United States Senate if there were no defined parliamentary process for making decisions! Constituency-based decisions of the medical staff are most frequently based on unanimous consensus rather than on business principles using sound operational policy. This can dramatically slow progress on a turnaround.

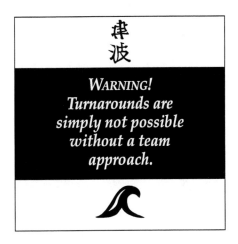

WARNING!
Turnarounds are simply not possible without a team approach.

■ *The motivation of the health professional is fundamentally different from that of the health administrator.* The difference in perspective between health professionals and administrators is particularly acute during a turnaround. Physicians, nurses, and others in the health care field are trained to deal with complexity by coordinating their responses to multiple, complex tasks through individual effort. These tasks could include research, clinical care, education, administration, and other roles in the health care setting.

Administrators, on the other hand, respond to complexity in the health care environment by defining responsibilities, differentiating tasks, and following work activities through a series of interdependent accountabilities. The result is that health providers are viewed as lone rangers by administrators and that administrators are viewed as bureaucrats by health providers.

The problem of fundamental differences in perspective between clinicians and administrators is often confounding to turnaround leaders in health care. As an example, the physician often delivers state-of-the-art care with excellent outcomes and results in an organization where systems and profitability that are required to support the physicians are in jeopardy and in need of a turnaround. Too frequently, physicians in such situations do not fully understand the principles of simultaneity, rapidity, complexity, uncertainty, management by intuition, and leader objectivity, which require turnaround leadership.

■ *Change-related strategies in the past related more to appeasement rather than collaboration.* Because the health care system has been flush with resources, it has been relatively easier to resolve opposition and conflict through deals, money, and other similar tools of appeasement. A turnaround scenario will not be successful unless it includes compromise and collaboration obtained through direct and open discussion. Collaboration requires active interaction, dialogue, and understanding of how increasingly scarce resources will be allocated. Such an approach is foreign to the health care industry and represents a unique challenge for the turnaround leader.

■ *Health professionals tend to identify more with their profession than with the organization with whom they are affiliated.* One of the key strategies for survival in health care is integration. Turnaround situations will no doubt require consideration of integration models. The difficulty is that most health professionals have as much or more allegiance to their professional organizations and societies as they do to organizations. After all, the rewards of the professions are often derived from peers, not organizations. One of the challenges for the turnaround leader is to align health professionals' interests with those of the organization.

■ *Too much focus is directed at control rather than the viability of the organization.* Because of the inherent distrust that exists between providers and health care institutions, there is often considerable energy and focus placed on who is in control! This is due to high levels of fear and anxiety associated with the turbulence and uncertainty surrounding our health care system. The health care world senses the coming of the tsunami. Some want to build bigger dikes. Others concentrate on building bigger bridges. Still others want to focus on the drainage systems. And still others are finding refuge in new environments. All of these conflicting opinions about where to focus energy require discussions about who is in control! The difficulty is that too little discussion is focused on future viability and in preparing for the tsunami.

CHAPTER X

The Philosophical Triad and Organizational Culture

The Cornerstone of the Turnaround

"If you are going to change something, you've got to live on vision before you live on reality. You have to be so inspired by the vision that you keep telling everybody until it gets in them, and they start living it with you."

Father Michael Scanlon

The Essence of Reason

Charles Bragg is an infamous artist whose paintings often depict the dilemmas of real life in interesting and provocative ways. One of his more interesting paintings is a picture of a gnome holding a chicken by the neck in one hand and a cracked egg in the other. The title of the painting is "Which Comes First?" The question of which comes first is at the core of culture. Is it vision? Or mission? Or values? Although the principle of simultaneity may apply, we consider the definition of vision a critical first step in starting the turnaround.

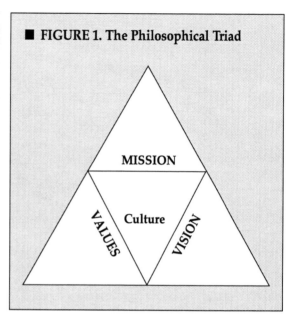

■ FIGURE 1. The Philosophical Triad

MISSION

VALUES   Culture   VISION

The First Step

Jonathan Swift in 1711 stated: "Vision is the art of seeing things invisible." Vision—without it, a turnaround is not possible! A clearly defined vision is central to the process of effective management of a turnaround. Nanus defines a vision as "composed of one part foresight, one part insight, plenty of imagination and judgment, and often a healthy dose of chutzpah. It occurs to a well-informed open mind, a mind prepared by a lifetime of learning and experience, one sharply attuned to emerging trends and developments in the world outside the organization."[1]

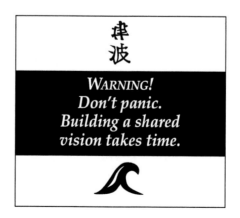

WARNING!
Don't panic.
Building a shared
vision takes time.

Once the vision is defined, it is important not only to share it with all key staff and senior management but also to communicate it widely throughout the entire organization. Buy-in or commitment to the vision can only be harnessed if it is heard, discussed, debated, and considered by everyone. Alignment with the vision will occur naturally if it is held in front of the organization every working day. So let's be clear—what are we trying to create?

The vision creates a template that allows everyone in the organization to measure the progress of the turnaround. It forces accountability in an environment filled with anxiety and trepidation by serving as the anchor. By focusing on the future, the staff, the board, and other critical stakeholders are prevented from becoming stuck in the inevitable blame-setting and negativity associated with the organization's decline and current situation.

The vision statement should never be hung on the wall and forgotten. A real vision serves as the framework for the leader's thinking and actions. To be effective, the leader must find ways to make people live by the vision statement, to make it real. Use the vision frequently and publicly. Incorporate it into the performance evaluation of all employees by asking:

A Vision...

- Creates a compelling picture of how we see the organization in the future compared to the present.
- Invigorates the staff and other key stakeholders to take risks with leadership in the turnaround process.
- Expresses our optimism, values, and hope about what the organization can become.
- Is a beacon of direction for navigating the tumultuous waters of a tsunami.
- Portrays an obtainable and attractive future for the organization.
- Exposes the organization and its people to the future in ways that have not been previously considered.
- Is not an architectural plan but a plea of the heart in defining where to go.
- Speaks to the organization, not to the industry.
- Is slightly embarrassing!

- How have you contributed to the fulfillment of our new organizational vision during the past year?
- What changes have you initiated in the organization or in yourself that have contributed to the fulfillment of our new vision?

Remember, without a clear vision, a turnaround is simply not possible.

The Next Step

The mission statement is considered the foundation of the traditional strategic plan for an organization. It is a description of the reason for being for the organization and is often used to help gain support for the organization from internal and external stakeholders. The existing mission in a turnaround situation inevitably becomes obsolete because of the fundamental changes that are required in the organization's purposes and reason for being.

Reestablishing a new organizational mission has an important impact on the staff during a turnaround, because it:

■ Reconnects them to a new sense of purpose.

■ Creates a starting place for them on the journey toward the organization's vision.

■ Produces an appropriate tension between where they are and where they need to go if the turnaround is to be successful.

In writing a new mission statement for the organization:

■ Review all old mission-related documents to assess their relevance to the turnaround situation.

■ Include a clear statement about the new organization's purpose, stakeholders, and strategy.

■ Allow a broad base of external stakeholders and staff to review and have input into the mission statement.

■ Display the completed mission statement prominently throughout the organization, including lobbies, your calendar book, and in plastic holders on tables at board meetings.

■ Keep the mission statement to no more than one page.

■ Don't include anything in your mission statement that you are unwilling to back up with action.

Aspects of the mission statement to consider include:

■ What are our basic purposes?

■ What is unique or distinctive about our organization?

■ Who are our principal customers, clients, or users?

■ What are our principal services—present or future?

■ What are the major market segments or niches of our organization?

■ How does our business differ today from five years ago?

■ Are there certain philosophical issues that are important to our organization?

■ What special considerations do we have regarding the board of directors? The general public? Legislative bodies? Employees and employers? Other health care providers?

■ What role does our organization want to play in the broader health care system of our community?

The Last Step

Establish the values—the essence of our beliefs. The importance of values relates to the potential for organizational tension to evolve where disparity exists between workers, leadership, and governance. Confluence in values among these three organizational stakeholders creates a synergy that will make success in the turnaround likely. The leader of the turnaround has a particularly important role in facilitating the evolution of organizational values.

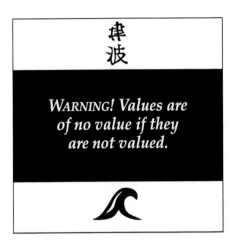

> **WARNING!** *Values are of no value if they are not valued.*

One of the first steps in a turnaround situation is to fully understand the current values of the organization. The understanding is often shared in quiet and intimate ways rather than through formal channels. In many cases, the rhetoric does not meet the reality! So, what are the best ways for determining the existing corporate values? There are certain methods that we believe can be important in helping the turnaround leader determine existing values:

- *Listen to the stories of the organization.* The stories that are shared about people, events, successes, and failures often provide the best clues on the real values of the organization.

- *Observe behavior.* Espoused values and behavior are frequently incongruent. In many turnaround situations, senior staff will often espouse a team philosophy that includes office posters trumpeting the need to work together! The stress and strain of the turnaround process, however, makes them protective of turf, resistant to new thinking, and suspicious of open communication.

- *Share among workers.* If the leader of a turnaround situation extends an open philosophy to ideas, thoughts, and perspectives early in the turnaround process, he or she will often be the recipient of information from many divergent sources. The information is often unfiltered and provides an unparalleled opportunity to assess the true values of the organization.

Values, once articulated, can be a powerful force in carrying the turnaround process forward. Each leader and each worker brings his or her own set of values to a turnaround situation. In establishing organizational values, the process must include an examination of each key participant's personal values. In particular, a dysynchrony between the values of the leader and the values of the workers will undermine the turnaround. Examples in recent years include:

■ Many medical schools in recent years have hired deans who espoused primary care, a community-based value that flies in the face of the specialty, quaternary care traditions of academic medical centers. The result: Deans don't last!

■ The leader of a managed care initiative values the need for a collaborative, team-oriented approach to health care involving the application of a care *management* philosophy. Care management is defined as the provision of a comprehensive, locally accessible, patient-focused continuum of care that improves the health status of a population served by a health care organization. The values of the organization dictate that physicians be controlled through contractual and financial constraints. Governance does not include their perspective. The result: The managed care initiative fails!

■ Turnarounds call for a high degree of openness and flexibility on the part of participants. A leader is selected who espouses those values but who, in reality, is defensive when confronted. The result: Workers disinvest themselves from the turnaround process!

A final comment is important. In the formative stage of the turnaround, agreed-upon values may be more rhetoric than real. This problem is especially pronounced in a turnaround situation. To rectify the incongruity between articulated values and real values, it is essential for the leader who desires a change in organizational values to live them day in and day out. Without the leader's commitment to the values, the rhetoric will become the reality.

The philosophical triad of the turnaround process involves the interrelation of vision, mission, and values. Furthermore, at the core of the philosophical and operational triads resides the organizational culture. The core of the turnaround effort is based on the culture of the organization. The complexity in understanding the impact of culture revolves around the dynamics of the old and new cultures, which interface in a turnaround situation.

As turnaround efforts unfold, a new culture will emerge and evolve as the standard for sustaining the organization into the future. Clearly, everyone must be cognizant of and invested in the new culture. More important, however, is the actual process of creating a culture, which evolves from actions, words, and deeds.

In addition to establishing a new culture, it is equally important to fully understand and appreciate the old culture (i.e., pre-tsunami). The turnaround leaders must never forget how ingrained the patterns of culture can become in an organization.

Each component of the operational and philosophical triads contributes to the overall organizational culture in unique and disparate ways. The culture, in addition to the contribution of these components, is composed of several key elements:

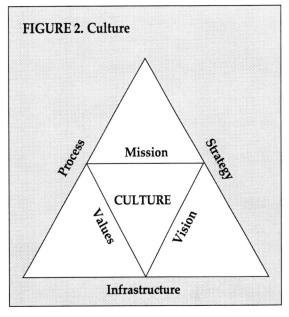

FIGURE 2. Culture

■ **Norms.** The ground rules for behavior in the organization must often be reset in a turnaround situation. The traditional artifacts and guides for normative behavior are often barriers to the turnaround. An example of a health care norm that cannot be tolerated in a turnaround is automatic deference to the physician. While important to the overall turnaround process in health care, physicians as a group are not necessarily in the best position for determining future directions. Physician executives have an especially important role in revising the norm so that physicians become a constructive part of a team.

■ **Assumptions.** Every organization has either invented, discovered, or developed ways of coping with internal and external threats. The turnaround often threatens the core assumptions of the organization and poses a challenge to the traditional way members have learned to respond. An example of a classic assumption made by many health care entities is that capitation will not enter the marketplace. The organizational behavior then reverts to stalling and ignoring tactics that ultimately fail, precipitating *The Turnaround Imperative.*

■ **Rules.** The spoken and unspoken frameworks for surviving the organizational game constitute the rules of culture. Newcomers must "learn the ropes" to succeed. Rules that are counter to the turnaround must be considered, addressed, and revised. Examples of rules in health care that are obstacles to successful turnarounds include overinflating the budget because it will be cut by 50 percent anyway and paying lip service to planning but doing your own thing once group plans are set.

■ **Climate.** The climate is conveyed through the physical layout of the organization and the way in which members interact with customers or other outside stakeholders. Examples include ease of admission to the outpatient setting, the maze of hallways that must be traversed in order to obtain a simple laboratory or radiological procedure, and the way patients are treated when calling the institution, which may include rudeness, multiple transfers, long hold periods, or inability to hear a real human voice! Climate is one of the most important elements in meeting customer satisfaction and, yet, one of the most frequently ignored in health care.

Each of the six components—infrastructure, process, strategy, vision, mission, and values—surrounding the core of organizational culture represent key considerations for the turnaround effort. An integrated approach that considers all components is absolutely necessary. Concentrating energy in any one area to the exclusion of others will undermine the turnaround effort and the development of a new organization.

References

1. Nanus, B. *Visionary Leadership*. San Francisco, Calif.: Jossey-Bass Publishers, 1992

2. Shein, E. *Organizational Culture and Leadership*. San Francisco, Calif.: Jossey-Bass Publishers, 1985.

CHAPTER XI

Creating Sustainable Momentum: The Importance of People, Process, and Places

"The change of motion is proportional to the motive force impressed; and is made in the direction of the right line in which that force is impressed."

Sir Isaac Newton
Philosophiae Naturalis Principia

Preparing for the Next Tsunami

Health care tsunamis are about to hit shore. They will be catastrophic events, disasters. Tsunamis represent uncontrolled change in the face of tradition and fixed paradigms. The measure of success in responding to the tsunami of change that will wash over health care during this decade is whether or not health care leaders will be successful at establishing sustainable momentum for their organizations' future.

Organizations that have ignored the warning signs of the impending tsunami and that have been involved only in developmental change are exceptionally susceptible to devastation. As discussed in Chapter II, developmental change is incremental in nature and improves on what is. A developmental change response cannot adequately prepare the organization for the radical change needed in a turnaround situation.

A developmental change response preserves the organization's status quo while moving the organization incrementally ahead. It represents the major methodology for planning in the health care industry during the 1970s. Although there is a desire on the part of many sectors of the health care industry to continue a developmental approach, these responses will be insufficient for dealing with the coming tsunami. Examples include:

■ Physicians who believe that solo practice will continue despite a general corporatization of health care and who refuse to engage in active managed care practices will be out of business.

■ Academic medical centers that refuse to engage their providers on the importance of cost-effective care despite the quality of their product will find no bidders.

■ Organizations that cannot provide a truly integrated continuum of care will be unsuccessful in providing managed care for the Medicare population. The failure to establish systems for providing care to one-third of the population creates an untenable method of health care delivery.

Organizations that have engaged in strategic changes while they were better off are still highly susceptible to substantial damage from the coming tsunami. The issue involves the pace of change. Strategic change by definition is planned and methodical. It moves the organization from the old state to a new state over a controlled period. In general, there is no immediate crisis during a strategic change process.

The coming tsunami requires a dramatic, unplanned, and sustained response to a shifting environment. A strategic approach, while useful in the traditional environment, is an insufficient investment in the rapid destructive phase of the tsunami wave.

The only organizations that *may* experience only slight damage are those engaged in transformational change. Recognition that a tsunami is coming is the first predictor of survival. Building on higher ground, with different groups of people using different structures that employ different technologies, will prevent the type of destruction that will inevitably be experienced by most of the health care system. However, it does not create immunity from *The Turnaround Imperative.*

The result is that all of us in health care will experience the ravages of the tsunami! Some organizations are seemingly unaware of the coming events. Others are aware but unprepared. Still others welcome the change.

If your organization survives the tsunami, it must be prepared to respond to the natural aftermath. All of the preceding chapters have outlined processes and strategies for implementing an effective turnaround. Although these steps are crucial in initiating a turnaround effort, they are insufficient for creating sustainable momentum.

Creating sustainable momentum requires shifting gears to a different level, to a different pace and process, to a different leadership style. We believe that sustaining transformational change over long periods is exceedingly difficult for organizations and individuals. The emotional burnout and trauma inherent in radical change eventually take their toll on the human resources of the organization. At that point, an organization can either discard human resources or move toward developing sustainable momentum. The considerations required to achieve sustainable momentum include:

Change Management. As noted previously, the formative stage of a turnaround situation involves transformational change. Once the turnaround moves beyond the initial crisis and rebuilding stage to the sustainable stage, other approaches to change become more applicable for the turnaround leader.

Change management is a cornerstone for creating sustainable momentum and eventually requires moving the organization back toward a more strategic approach from a transformational process. Rather than engaging in simultaneous activities, the organization uses a structured approach. Intended chaos is replaced by planned considerations. Power becomes an insufficient lever and must be replaced with collaboration. The dramatic is modified with measured approaches. Movement of the organization on the change continuum toward a more strategic approach results in sustainable momentum.

The art of leadership in *The Turnaround Imperative* is especially important in managing the change process. It is as important to recognize the need for moving toward a transformational response as it is to recognize the need for the measured responses inherent in strategic change. The ability to move the organization from one part of the change continuum to another at the appropriate time helps create sustainable momentum.

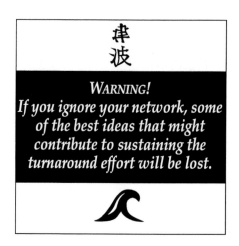

WARNING!
If you ignore your network, some of the best ideas that might contribute to sustaining the turnaround effort will be lost.

Continuous Networking. The best information in a fast-changing environment is not from books or articles. The very best information comes from colleagues. Participation in a network, from our perspective, can be one of the most valuable, although time-intensive, activities for the turnaround leader. Networks can range from informal gatherings of colleagues facing similar situations to formal participation in organization activities designed to assist the leader.

Scanning should be required by staff at all levels, not just for the leader. New ideas, new methods, new relationships, and new information sources are all critical parts of creating sustainable momentum. For example, how many health care organizations are actively surfing the Internet for validation, information, and idea exchange. We suspect very few. In an environment demanding constant change, harvesting the network can be your route to survival.

Leadership Style. In Chapter V, the leadership requirements of the formative stage of *The Turnaround Imperative* are described. To foster sustainable momentum, however, a different style is needed by the leader.

■ *Leadership must be shared between the leader, the followers, and governance.* Unlike the formative stages of the turnaround where, in many cases, the leader needed to act in an autonomous manner, the movement toward sustainable momentum requires a collaborative leadership style. In our estimation, the transition from the authoritarian leadership style needed in the formative stages to the collaborative leadership style of sustainable momentum is the most difficult task for the turnaround leader. The change is difficult from two perspectives.

First, the turnaround leader must alter his or her style to engage in behaviors that may be diametrically opposed to the effective styles in the formative stages. Second, the individual members of the senior management team and of the workforce grow accustomed to the style required in the formative stages and resist movement toward a more collaborative leadership style. As an example, early in a turnaround the leader frequently must make decisions without adequate information. Later, as the organization becomes more stable, the turnaround leader will continue to be placed in the role of decision maker, even if he or she attempts to move the decisions to other individuals in the organization.

Movement toward a collaborative leadership style is important for several reasons:

- Personal survival dictates the need for a change in style.
- Staff members have developed to a point where the vision is ingrained and much of the old behaviors have dissipated.
- The organization will benefit from more thoughtful, broad-based, multi-disciplinary decisions.
- Failure to change will result in the leader's being viewed as an autocrat, with all of the problems associated with such a style.

Turnaround Leadership Styles

Formative Stage	Sustainable Momentum Stage
Authoritarian	Collaborative
Pressed	Metered
Independent action	Team-oriented action
High profile	Shared profile
Personal sacrifice	Personal nurturance
Directive	Empowerment
Sprinter	Long-distance runner

- *Nurturing mind, body, and spirit becomes very important.* The personal toll on the turnaround leader can be very substantial because of the pressures experienced during the formative stage. Frequently, the turnaround leader puts aside his or her self-interests in favor of those of the organization. To survive on a long-term basis, the leader must transition with the organization as it moves in a sustainable momentum stage. We recommend an extended vacation, a course of study unrelated to work or professional responsibilities, or a rediscovery of personal interests and hobbies.

- *Delegate decisions and authority to the appropriate level.* In the formative stage of the turnaround, the leader often maintains an exceptionally high degree of visibility in decision making, in problem solving, and in representing the organization. Sustainable momentum requires sharing these responsibilities throughout the organization. An extension of collaborative leadership is empowerment of the organization!

■ *Speed is a vital factor, but it requires the pace of a long-distance runner.* Unlike the sprint of the formative stage, movement toward sustainable momentum allows the "luxury" of engaging in a more strategic and developmental change response. A metered rather than an urgent investment of time and energy takes the organization into a more rational frame of reference as change continues.

Furthermore, organizations need respite as much as individuals. The rapid pace, chaotic process, mandatory methods, and dramatic change inherent in the formative stage simply tire everyone! Just as individual leaders must "take a break," so must the organization modify its behaviors to make the transition to sustainable momentum.

Leadership Capacity. The investment in leadership development is often underappreciated and undervalued in the health care industry. In the post-tsunami stage, development of new leaders who can manage the new environment is absolutely essential. The focus of the turnaround process is frequently on the leader of the effort. Creating sustainable momentum requires moving from an individual leadership model to one that fosters shared leadership at all levels within the organization.

As an example, the turnaround leader must recognize the physician leadership involvement will be crucial in the future health care organization. However, most physicians are ill-equipped to serve in a governance capacity in a large health care corporation. The patterns of physician involvement in health care have traditionally involved advocacy for their individual or their group's needs. The fiduciary responsibilities of participation in governance of large health care enterprises, however, require a different mentality and level of participation by physicians.

So, how can it be accomplished? There are several approaches to leadership development that are tried and true. The turnaround leader has an especially important role in mentoring new leaders for the organization. Traditionally, many organizations have invested heavily in both formal and informal education of the workforce. One of the best ways for developing leadership is by providing the opportunity for new and evolving leaders to exhibit their capabilities. Finally, health care organizations frequently do not offer sufficient rewards for individuals who engage in leadership activities. Rewarding leadership behavior is absolutely essential to sustaining the organization's evolution.

In essence, the challenge of the turnaround leader is to develop the requisite leadership at all levels of the organization. Without such efforts, the needed stabilization of the organization will not be sustained.

Cultivate People. It is important to recognize that not everyone is a leader. Just as it is important to support leaders, so is it imperative that organizations serious about moving toward sustainable momentum engage in activities to cultivate human resources. The redevelopment and growth of an organization following a tsunami will often outpace the growth of individuals in the organization. The tsunami event will precipitate clearer divisions among people within the organization, separating those who are capable of managing change from those who cannot keep pace. The ability to recognize the difference between those two types of employees makes the critical difference in building sustainable momentum.

Turnover of the organizational workforce in the post-tsunami state is to be anticipated. The turnaround leader's role is to help clarify for those hanging on after the tsunami whether or not they should stay. It is important to offer gentle but direct and clear advice to members of the workforce on their potential contributions to the new organization. This activity is often the most difficult part of the turnaround process. It is important to work with the human resource department and the performance appraisal system to enable the leader to give appropriate feedback and evaluations to employees regarding other opportunities.

Turnover of staff can be one of the most helpful mechanisms for the leader to establish new energy, commitment, and focus within the organization. New hires in the post-tsunami stage have not experienced the pain of the turnaround. Furthermore, they do not bring old baggage to the table as the new organization builds sustainable momentum.

For those individuals who survive the tsunami and adapt to the new environment, an equal amount of support is required from organizational leadership. Cultivating the skills, abilities, and talents of this group is as important as all other activities related to creating sustainable momentum.

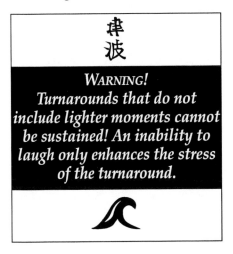

WARNING!
Turnarounds that do not include lighter moments cannot be sustained! An inability to laugh only enhances the stress of the turnaround.

Team Development. The health care system of the past has been based on the premise that the solitary activities of the physician, the administrator, the nurse, or the hospital can meet the needs of the individual patient. The model worked in a fee-for-service environment, but the world has changed. Now the demands of accelerated information management, the increasing complexity of service delivery, and the evolving fixed payment structures all require a more team-oriented approach to the delivery of health care.

In fact, many organizations are moving toward the development of their systems as *care management organizations.* The care management organization is an integrated health care organization that provides a comprehensive, patient-focused continuum of care through the appropriate application of services and the active participation of providers, staff, and management as a team in clinical, quality, and financial processes inherent in providing value to customers.

Many barriers exist in successful implementation of a team approach to health care. Competition between providers, inadequate communication, differences in resource availability between various members of the health care team, and other similar characteristics interfere with team development. To build a team, the turnaround leader must:

- Assemble the right membership.
- Establish a common goal.
- Create appropriate ground rules to facilitate effectiveness of the group.
- Foster mutuality of trust and respect of team members.
- Implement effective communication mechanisms.
- Establish norms for interaction.
- Understand how to appreciate and utilize individual differences among group members.
- Teach everyone how to manage team processes.
- Create a norm of self-monitoring and self-evaluation on the part of the team.

Movement toward sustainable momentum requires a much deeper team commitment and a high degree of mutuality. The transition will be as difficult for members of the team as the transition from authoritarian to collaborative leadership is for the leader. An investment in team development at this point in the turnaround cycle should be considered.

Workable Organizational Structure. Moving beyond the trauma of the turnaround state requires attention to organizational structure. The free-flowing, man-the-lifeboats mentality that dominates the immediate post-tsunami stage must be modified to a more functional approach to create sustainable momentum.

The structure of the organization must be continuously reevaluated following the initial turnaround. Frequently, the structure created in the formative stage of the turnaround must be altered as a more stable environment evolves.

Finally, the roles of individuals in the early stages of the turnaround may differ markedly from the roles of these individuals in later stages. It is important to recognize that role modification must be actively pursued, because some roles important in a turnaround are not conducive to the maintenance of sustainable momentum.

Invest Properly. There are three key investments for the future of health care. Too often, attention is given to financial investments and inadequate attention is devoted to the other elements. Investments in human capital are required. The people of the organization, as noted throughout this book, are the key to survival in a turnaround situation. Appropriate and timely investments in people will make the difference between success and failure of the turnaround effort.

A key systems investment is in the area of information. The resources of the health care system have been traditionally invested in infrastructure. In today's health care environment, access to timely and reliable information will create sustainable momentum.

Appropriate Change Methodologies. The past several years have seen a plethora of books and articles espousing the need for reengineering, total quality management, continuous quality improvement, and a host of other strategies designed to enhance organizational effectiveness. *The Turnaround Imperative* may require implementation of one or more of these change methodologies. At the least, we believe that the adoption of one or several of these processes is essential for creating sustainable momentum.

Organizations that are successful in the post-tsunami stage will find ways to continue integrating these processes with the existing structure, culture, and management philosophy. Sustainable momentum cannot be a reality without the application of these change methodologies. Why?

■ Payers are demanding value through access to higher quality services at lower cost.

■ The regulatory environment now requires adoption of improvement processes for purposes of accreditation.

■ By their nature, these processes force an organization to continually evaluate its effectiveness in a changing environment.

■ Adoption of these methodologies prepares the organization to more effectively move from transformational to strategic and developmental change and back again as the environment dictates. The organization's ability to cope with more tsunamis is markedly improved.

Effective Communication. Too frequently, organizations rely on formal, written communication as the sole method for conveying changes in the organization. Turnarounds by their very nature are dynamic and interactive. In addition to written communication, the turnaround leader must provide ample opportunity for the senior management team and others in the organization to engage in dialogue and strategic thinking.

Retreats, as noted previously, are a common method for engaging individuals in the turnaround. However, once the formative stages of the turnaround pass, these sessions frequently are held on an annual basis. To continue sustainable momentum and to help senior managers cope with the dynamic environment of the ongoing turnaround process, other forums are needed.

Specifically, one- or two-day quarterly retreats with key members of the management team will greatly assist in sustaining the turnaround effort. When you've gone through a period of dramatic change, it is important to step back now and then to continue the process of refocusing, reconnecting,, and reenergizing the team through a more strategic approach. The quarterly forum or retreat offers the senior management team the opportunity to reflect on the changes in style needed to move the organization forward after the immediate post-tsunami period.

Celebrate Successes. In the heat of the turnaround, celebration is often neglected because of the pace of change. A personalized outreach by the turnaround leader through informal interaction with the staff of the organization can have a markedly positive impact on morale. More important, the new organizational culture can foster self-sustaining momentum independent of the leader through ritual and celebration!

Celebratory events that sustain momentum within the organization can include:

- Recognition of achievement of goals and objectives important to the turnaround.
- Annual events that recognize the efforts of the workforce in the turnaround.
- Individual awards to people in the organization based on peer recognition for contributions to the turnaround effort.
- Opportunities for personal interaction and discussion with the organization's leadership on future directions.
- Informal gatherings that continue to reinforce and acknowledge progress toward realization of the turnaround.

CHAPTER XII

Health Care in
the Next Century

A Look Ahead Before You Get Behind

"I never make predictions, especially about the future."

Yogi Berra

Continuous Consideration of Tsunamis

The relative quiet of the early and mid-20th Century is in stark contrast to the last major period of tsunami waves. If we consider the late 19th Century, society experienced tsunami upon tsunami as part of the Industrial Revolution. A new era of tsunamis is upon us! Until we adjust, until we modify our thinking, until we can adapt to the new environment, society will experience wave upon wave of change.

Dealing with the present is difficult enough! So, why consider the future? Because, in our estimation, we have entered a period in which *continuous consideration of tsunamis* is essential to survival. Among the many changes occurring within our society, it appears that three particular changes will have a continuing and sustainable impact on the future of health care.

The Global Economy. Our world is increasingly interdependent. The transfer of credits and debits happens electronically with the entry of a code and a password. The use of money no longer occurs during the daylight hours of any one nation, but continuously, 24 hours a day, seven days a week. And our interdependence is accelerating. Such an environment serves as the nidus for continuous tsunamis.

Human Genome Project. Perhaps one of the most lasting contributions of our generation will be the results of the Human Genome Project. It is unleashing information; methodologies for detection, treatment, and prevention of illness; and the specter of intervention in the human experiment that did not seem possible 10 years ago. Aside from the ethical, political, social dimensions of the project, it will fundamentally alter our concept of "medicine" as we move into the 21st Century.

Information Age. Ten years ago, the idea of holding a tool in the palm of your hand that was as powerful as all the computers in existence 20 years earlier seemed impossible. Today, it is a reality. The speed of processing information is doubling about every 18 months! The consequence of such change will result in a chip or processing capability 512 times faster than today's environment. Unless a plateau is reach (which is deemed unlikely by computer experts), the reality of real-time information seems feasible. And real time information is only one step away from the capability of computer knowledge.

Gazing ahead is a risky business at best. Here are a few of our thoughts on what lies ahead over the next decade.

Evidence-based medicine. The specter of evidence-based medicine would not be feasible without the new technologies of the latest information systems. It promotes practice patterns based on specific outcomes data tied to specific problems. Likewise, the costs of services are linked to the investment of resources. As a result, it will push health care upstream toward more epidemiology-based approaches that alter the health status of populations rather than simply individuals. Evidence-based medicine is not tied to specific types of providers. Rather it allows the organization to deliver the services irrespective of provider type *if* the outcomes are comparable. For example, if the care of an acupuncturist can be shown to clearly augment the treatment of chronic fatigue syndrome or arthritis or migraine headache, it will be used as a standard course of treatment. It is the future of American medicine.

Outcomes accreditation. If one accepts the notion of evidence-based medicine, the possibility of outcomes accreditation is only an incremental step. Over the past century, medicine has developed a standard of peer assessment for entry into the profession. With the advent of information technologies, others with less comprehensive knowledge—but more expert technical skill—will be empowered to provide services. When Laennec invented the stethoscope, only physicians were allowed the opportunity to use the new tool. The same applies to the thermometer. In today's health care world, no one would even think of restricting such basic tools to a single profession. In a similar manner, the advent of the computer will push knowledge outward. Outcomes—not specific professional credentials—will become increasingly important. As a result, we will no doubt face the possibility of credentialing of the professions and institutions based on outcomes. The medical profession will fight it. Society will demand it.

Commodity-based pricing for services. Health care today involves a cost-based pricing strategy. The entire process of negotiation between health care providers and payers relates to the question of price. In the future, as prices are increasingly ratcheted down, there will be a point when prices are essentially equal. At that point, other factors will enter the equation in determining who provides health care. Where there is price equivalency, commodity-based pricing will take hold. Many health care organizations are at the initial stages of commodity pricing in certain cardiology services such as angioplasty and coronary artery bypass surgery. Like VCRs, like computers, like other commodity products, health care will enter an entirely new era of challenge. We are at the entry point of commodity-based pricing. It will be a reality within the next decade.

Consolidated delivery systems. Today, the industry is moving in a direction of greater and greater *integration*. While important, it is one step short of the eventual outcome, consolidated delivery systems. Integrated health care systems generally are restricted to the traditional elements of medicine and health care. Public health functions may not be considered. In consolidated delivery systems, comprehensive organizations will pursue strategies of sustainable health for the population served. Not only will these organizations be seamless, they will provide one-stop shopping for a variety of services, including social support systems, housing, community aid, and other health-related functions of our society. It is the next logical step in the evolution of health care systems.

Focus on health as an investment rather than an enterprise. As the United States is faced with increasing pressure on the allocation of scarce resources, it will force the health care enterprise to become more investment-oriented. An investment strategy, however, cannot work without the cooperation and active involvement of the individual. New strategies for engaging individuals in their health and well-being will be developed. Health promotion and wellness strategies will finally move beyond marketing hype to real investments in changing people's health status. Self-monitoring mechanisms will assist the individual in a continuous self-health assessment process. Health care cannot help but move in this direction. It is the imperative of economics.

Global health systems. Just as the world is shrinking, so will our scope expand! The cross-pollination of societies is accelerating at ever-increasing rates. The advent of the North American Free Trade Agreement (NAFTA) will precipitate the expansion of health enterprises into Mexico and Canada. Cross-border health services are becoming the norm for the southwest border states. Adoption of an American free trade initiative will expand the activity to South America. The Pacific Basin will tie itself together for a whole set of services that extend beyond traditional business relationships. In fact, U.S. health systems are already engaged in discussions about the delivery of care in Singapore, Saudi Arabia, Hong Kong, Australia, and other countries. The list expands on a daily basis. Global health systems will become major contributors to the American economy.

Extensive use of cyber-technology. Cyberspace is an illusive, yet increasingly real place. Shared access to data, real-time decision making, and distributed information resources are becoming the norm. Consultations are occurring via video-conference. Radiology films are being interpreted via fiberoptic connections. Two-way interactive discussions are occurring between physicians speaking different languages through the use of simultaneous interpretation that allows consultations to occur from any source in the world. The adoption of cyber-technology will allow health care organizations to move the actual delivery of service closer to the individual. No longer will we be restricted to specific locations that require the consumer to come to us! If we follow the flow of information, we will provide care in the home. It's only a matter of time.

Consumer control. The movement of information toward the consumer also changes the locus of control. Not only is this a trend, but it is crucial if we are to be successful in creating sustainable health. Responsibility will be returned to the consumer along with increased accountability. Employers are beginning to recognize the value of a healthy workforce. Incentivization of employees will accelerate the movement toward more personal accountability. Consumer control represents a cornerstone of future health care systems.

Professional movement from a guild-oriented priesthood to a socially accountable partner with consumers. As with the priests of yore, society has conferred upon medicine special rights and privileges in relating to people. The profession of medicine is based on a guild approach. It really isn't much different than the guilds of past centuries where members of the guild trained apprentices and passed on the special knowledge. Physicians and other health professionals go through special programs (medical/health education) sponsored by members of the guild (medical/health science schools). Clinician are given special training (residencies and fellowships) in special places (hospitals and clinics). At the end of the training (apprenticeship), they are allowed the opportunity to become recognized (licensed) for their special knowledge. The license allows them to perform certain functions on behalf of society. When the knowledge was held by the profession, such an approach was successful. As we move toward an era of distributed knowledge, the guild approach will no longer suffice. Managing these challenges will serve to redefine the role of health professions in society.

The next generation in health care will be an experience to behold. Surviving tsunamis involves all the elements discussed in this book. It is part science and part art. The challenge for the surfer of tsunamis is learning to balance on the wave of all waves. *The Turnaround Imperative* is upon us. Now is the time to prepare. Consider the alternatives. Best of luck!

GLOSSARY

Assumptions. A part of the organizational culture, core attitudes of the organization that are either invented, discovered, or developed as ways of coping with internal and external threats.

Care Management Organization. An integrated health care organization that provides a comprehensive, patient-focused continuum of care through the appropriate application of services and the active participation of providers, staff, and management as a team involved in clinical, quality, and financial processes inherent in providing value to customers.

Climate. A part of organizational culture, it conveys to individuals external to the organization the way it will interact with customers or other outside stakeholders.

Creators. Individuals in the organization who are committed to the sense of vision, strategy, and timing required for the successful turnaround. These people demonstrate their support through active involvement in all facets of the turnaround.

Developmental Change Response. An incremental change that improves on the present state and is prevalent in a secure and stable environment, most often occurring while the organization is in a dominant market position. It tends to preserve the status quo through maintenance of institutional prerogative, mission, and structure. Because it is not dramatic or threatening, a developmental change response is frequently understood, accepted, and embraced by followers. In predictable and sustainable environments, a developmental change response is a natural process that occurs under management with or without good leadership.

Formative Stage. The period immediately following a tsunami, early in the turnaround. It is characterized by chaos, confusion, devastation to existing systems and relationships, and the need for immediate action. The leadership style that predominates in the formative stage is authoritarian in nature.

Infrastructure. The core elements of an organization, including space, equipment, information and information systems, agreements and contracts, human resources, structure, and finances. Infrastructure is a critical component of the operational triad.

Mission. A description of the here and now situation for the organization. It is the foundation of the organization's current work.

Norms. As part of the culture, ground rules for behavior in the organization that serve as a guide for normative behavior.

Operational Triad. Integration of infrastructure, strategy, and process as an operational approach to the turnaround process.

Philosophical Triad. Inner core of the turnaround model that integrates vision, mission, and values of the organization.

Principle of Complexity. The principle evolves from requirements of the turnaround leader to contemporaneously manage the old organization and define a vision for the new entity. The leader must blend the two into a coherent framework for those who are assisting in creating the new order in a chaotic environment.

Principle of Management by Intuition. In situations demanding simultaneous, rapid decisions under complex and uncertain circumstances, there is a high need for intuitive thinking. The ability to see possibilities and patterns in the limited information available and to act on hunches is an important element of effective functioning as a leader in a turnaround situation (i.e., management by intuition).

Principle of Leader Objectivity. Impassioned objectivity is an absolute need on the part of the turnaround leader. Without it, the leader will succumb to old relationships, use of unreliable information, and existing paradigms of the organization facing a turnaround.

Principle of Rapidity. The principle notes that the simultaneous nature of the turnaround, coupled with the accelerated decision-making and change required, demands a unique leadership pace that cannot be sustained over protracted periods except through extra-human effort.

Principle of Simultaneity. The principle notes that multiple processes are occurring simultaneously and unpredictably, requiring flexibility on the part of the leader.

Principle of Uncertainty. Decisions in turnarounds are frequently ambiguous and generate uncertainty. The grey zone dominates turnaround decisions. The leader often is faced with pioneering new concepts for the organization that provide no guarantee of their effectiveness for the turnaround effort.

Process. The how of the turnaround, which includes attention to group dynamics, meeting flow, covert and overt resistance, behaviors, interpersonal relationships organizational norms, and other similar organizational dynamics.

Rules. As part of the culture, the spoken and unspoken framework for surviving the organizational game constitute the rules of culture.

Saboteurs. These are the ultimate turnaround busters! It is often impossible to negotiate any degree of support for the turnaround effort. Furthermore, they frequently cannot be trusted even when confronted directly about issues, concerns, or plans. They frequently become actively involved in opposition to the turnaround effort. These people are often the most difficult and time-consuming to manage. Ultimately, they can endanger the success of the turnaround.

Skeptics. These individuals hold strong divergent opinions about the need for the turnaround. They are often articulate adversaries who need more information before coming aboard the turnaround process.

Stabilization Stage. The point where vision, mission, values, strategy, process, and infrastructure have been clearly articulated for the organization. It is characterized by a more metered approach, clearer direction, a belief in its own survival on the part of the organization, and a renewed optimism about the future. The leadership style that predominates in the stabilization stage is collaborative in nature.

Strategic Change Response. A change that moves the organization from an old state to a new state and that can be articulated over a controlled period and, generally, when there is no crisis. The magnitude of change can be significant, unlike developmental change, and may involve altered organizational structures and directions. The strategic change response must possess leadership that understands and that is either in line with or ahead of outside forces.

Strategy. There are two elements of strategy inherent in the turnaround process, an internally and an externally focused activity. The first strategy element (internally focused) involves activities applied by the leader to the management of the turnaround process, such as identifying critical players, building team capacity, and assessing the organization's situation. The second element (externally focused) involves development of new strategic directions concerning the organization's future, such as defining new markets and articulating new programs and services. Both internally and externally focused elements of strategy are necessary for a successful turnaround.

Supporters. These people seem to be aligned with the stated vision and strategy and yet often are perceived as holding back their involvement in the turnaround.

Transformational Change Response. A change that forces the organization to reemerge after a period of chaos into a new state that is known during the initial phase of the change response. In a transformational change response, the organization evolves as part of an overall strategy.

Tsunami. A wave that emanates from a specific source, is not random, and is not related to wind. It's oceanic and never found in lakes. It's the largest type of wave known to mankind when it hits its destination. At sea, the tsunami often goes unnoticed. Unlike the ordinary wave, which, through its continuous action, rocks us about and erodes our confidence, the tsunami sweeps over the shoreline and destroys. After a tsunami hits, little remains the same.

Turnaround. A rapid organizational response involving multiple, simultaneous leadership activities and changes that will dictate the institution's future.

Turnaround Imperative. A last ditch effort to save an organization in a chaotic environment. It requires urgent and revolutionary responses, involving power and coercive strategies. Time is of the essence. A *priori*, it involves transformational change.

The Turnaround Model. Includes critical stakeholders (customers, governance, leadership, and management) that form a framework for considering two interrelated triads—the operational and the philosophical—with the culture of the organization at the core.

Vision. A compelling picture of the organization's future that can serve as a beacon of direction for navigating the tumultuous waters of a tsunami. The first dimension of vision involves the direction of the leader, which must be clear and compelling because, without a clear and compelling vision, neither the leader nor the organization can be sustained over time. The second dimension involves buy-in and investment by other stakeholders in the turnaround process.

Values. Values are the inherent approach of an organization to accomplishing its daily work. Values often dictate organizational response to problems, especially in periods of crisis.